A
MATERIA MEDICA

A MATERIA MEDICA.

Containing Provings and Clinical Verifications

OF

NOSODES AND MORBIFIC PRODUCTS.

BY

SAMUEL SWAN, M. D.

GYAN

Published by

Gyan Publishing House
5, Ansari Road
Daryaganj, New Delhi-110002
Phone: 011-47034999, 9811692060
E-mail: books@gyanbooks.com

Distribution Network
gyanbooks.com
India, USA, Canada, UK, Australia

ISBN: 978-93-6280-372-6 (HB)
First Published, 1888

2nd Impression 2024

Printed at: Gyan Press, Delhi.

A MATERIA MEDICA
Author: SAMUEL SWAN

A MATERIA MEDICA.

CONTAINING PROVINGS AND CLINICAL VERIFICATIONS

OF

NOSODES AND MORBIFIC PRODUCTS.

BY

SAMUEL SWAN, M. D.

NEW YORK:
PRESS OF PUSEY & CO.,
1398 BROADWAY.
1888.

This first Fascicle of a Materia Medica is placed before the profession as a feeler—if the demand for it shows that it meets a "long-felt want," the publication will be continued—if not this will be the first and the last.

INTRODUCTION TO PATHOGENESIS OF SACCHARUM LACTIS.

By SAMUEL SWAN, M. D.,
NEW YORK.

(*From " The Organon," Vol. III, Jan.*, 1880.)

THERE is something marvellous in the fact that drugs are made more potent by attenuation; but it is still more wonderful that substances, supposed to be inert in their crude state, should be rendered actively medicinal by the same process. But the degree of effective action is not a fixed fact, inherent in any particular degree of attenuation, but is dependent in its manifestation upon the *individual sensitiveness* of the person proving it, or the patient to whom it has been given. Thus, when homœopathically prescribed, in one case, a few grains of the crude drug will effect a cure; in another it will have no effect, but a low attenuation will cure ; while experience has shown that often, when a lower attenuation is powerless, a much higher will effect a rapid cure. A beautiful illustration of this last fact is recorded in *The Organon*, vol. ii., pp. 511-12, where it will be seen that a rapid cure was effected by *Carbo-veg.* 4 M, after the same in low dilution, and even in the 200th, had been of no avail. Some physicians are waiting till they know all about high potencies before they use them. They think they know all about the 30th or 200th, but all they really know about them is, that *they act.* If, instead of ventilating their mathematics by a long display of calculations, they were honestly to try a high potency of *the truly Homœopathic remedy* in a clearly defined case, they would never write more regarding the how and why.

There is scarcely an article of food that to some one has not proved a poison ; and there are poisons that have been and are constantly taken with apparent impunity. As an instance of the former, I will mention the case of poisoning by *Sugar* recorded in *The Organon*, vol. ii., p. 444. There are physicians who never prescribe a remedy on *one* proving; but as all these symptoms were cured with

Sac.-officinalis 10 M, 5 M, and 41 M, I accepted it as a proving, and have verified the correctness of the symptoms in my practice. The above is commended to the notice of the Boston University Medical School, who made a wonderful proving of *Sac.-lac.*, and congratulate them on having so many sensitive provers; and as they had many of the symptoms repeated while proving *Carb.-veg.* 3 trit., it shows conclusively that these provers were more susceptible to *Sac.-lac.* than to *Carb.-veg.* These symptoms, experienced after taking *Sac.-lac.*, are of value, and should be carefully noted. Again, in *The Organon*, vol. ii., pp. 286-87, is recorded a case of poisoning by *Milk*, which was cured with *Lac.-vaccinum* 10 M, ; and another case is given by Dr. Brooks in the *Medical Investigator*, vol. ix., p. 512. Call these articles by any other name than *Sugar* and *Milk*, and they would be accepted as very respectable poisons. My cases were cured by the same substances, highly attenuated, they becoming by that process so dissimilar in physical properties as not to be identified with the crude article by any known test, except that of the sensitive human organism; but, by that test, proving their similarity by curing the patients so that they could subsequently use sugar and milk, respectively, with impunity. "Scientific men," says a writer, "cannot admit that a degree of attenuation, beyond that in which can be found a molecure of the original drug, can contain any medicinal power peculiar to the drug from which it is made." But when such an attenuation is given in a case of sickness, having symptoms similar to those which inhere to the drug as evidenced by poisoning, and a cure results, not in one but in many cases, what other inference can be drawn than that the attenuation *does* contain *somewhat* of its original source, even though that *somewhat* connot be discovered by the most delicate physical or chemical tests.

But it is said, "Do you not potentize the sugar of milk in diluting a trituration, and will not it therefore modify the action of the drug, if it also possesses medicinal powers?" Certainly; the 30th dilution of the third trituration of *Calcarea* is a dilution of the *Calcarea* plus the *Sac.-lac.*; but it has been proved as a unit, and must be prescribed and considered as a unit, just as we use *Opium* as a unit, in spite of its multiplex composition. On the other hand, if it be asked whether the *crude* sugar of milk with which a substance is triturated, or which may be employed in dispensing a medicine, will not interfere with the action thereof, if the above statements are accurate, I would say, "Try for yourselves;" I have used Smith's 30th centesimal triturations, and always found that their action was that of the drug, and not of the sugar of milk, because probably very few would be, like the Boston provers, more sensitive to the latter than the former. *In this varying sensitiveness of individuals to different potencies and different drugs lay the entire failure of the Milwaukee Test.*

The belief or disbelief concerning the action of high potencies affects only the individual. If a physician is a believer in their efficacy, it is *only* because he has *tried* them, and can give his *own experience* for his belief. If another disbelieves, and will not try them for himself, and still denounces them and those who use them, he will most surely gravitate to Eclecticism, or possibly retrograde to Allopathy.

HAHNEMANN used sugar of milk as the most inert substance he could find. It was because of this supposed inertness, and on account of my belief that there is no substance so inert as not to show medicinal powers when attenuated, that the following proving of *Saccharum-lactis* was made.

PATHOGENESIS OF SACCHARUM LACTIS.

(The sign o signifies a merely *cured* symptom ; * signifies a pathogenetic symptom *also verified by a cure.* The figures immediately following a symptom denote the *authority* ; those in round brackets denote the *days* on which the symptom occurred; those in square brackets the *potency ;* r signifies *right ;* l signifies *left.*)

AUTHORITIES.

1. Miss M. Morgan, æt. 21.
2. B. Fincke, M.D.
3. Miss Julia Morgan,
4. E. W. Berridge, M.D.
5. Samuel Swan, M.D.
6. Mrs. Camm, M.D.
7. Mrs. Burritt, M.D.
8. E. A. Boardman, M.D.
9. Wm. Eggert, M.D.
10. J. A. Biegler, M.D.
11. Laura Morgan, M.D.

The provings by Nos. 1, 6, and 7 were made with the 200 cent. (Fincke), that of No. 3 with the 10 M (Fincke). The other provers took potencies made by Dr. Swan.

Miss Morgan commenced her proving at 9 a.m., May 25th, 1871, just before menses; she took drop doses of 200 every hour for one or two days.

The first effect appeared within an hour. Previous to the proving she was in perfect health. She had symptoms for two or three years. The omission of several hundred days is due to her discontinuing to take notes; she was so annoyed at the persistence of the symptoms, that she only resumed her notes after great persuasion. Dr. Fincke made provings on two ladies; one took two drops of 30th, the other took three drops of 53 M, The symptoms from 30th are here marked 2 A. Two symptoms marked [30] seem to be from another proving.

Mind and Disposition.

Sensation as if it were only by a great effort that she kept together, and would be much relieved if she could fall to pieces; she threw herself down for that purpose. 1 (19).

Loses her way in well-known streets; gets completely bewildered; walked from Fifth to Tenth Avenue while intending to go to Second Avenue; wondered how the avenue had got on the wrong side of the city. 1 (37.)

Imagines that there is a large hole in her back, just above sacrum; leans body back, and puts her hand there to fill it up. 1 (39).

Imagined that her mother wanted to kill her; kept constantly looking round to see if she was coming up behind her. 1 (49).

Imagines all day that some one is behind her. 1 (56).

After retiring, imagined that some one was under the bed; could not rest till she had looked. 1 (71).

Felt afraid to go to bed without looking under, over, and in everything. 1 (72).

Extremely nervous, jumps from her seat at the least unusual noise. 1 (49).

° Intense nervousness, seems as if she would fly out of her skin; wakes at 3 a.m., and does not sleep again till 7 a.m.; worries about all sorts of things; after 1 M slept quietly and soundly till 7 a.m., with entire relief from nervousness. 5.

10. She was taken suddenly with fear and trembling of the whole body, as from fright. 2 (1 after 3½ hours).

She thought she was young again, and that she wanted something which she feared she could not obtain. 2 (1).

Longing and melancholy as if home-sick, with oppressed breathing. 2 (1).

Awoke feeling very wretched and miserable, no particular pain. 6 (2).

Feeling of grievance and neglect, and as if her old long-forgotten troubles were brought back to her. 2 (1).

Her heart aches as if it would burst, yet she cannot weep. 2 (1).

The melancholy mood gradually lessens. 2 (3).

° The habitual sighing disappeared. 2 (6).

In forenoon a condition of melancholy and sadness as previously, but less, followed by burning and painfulness in l. mamma and nipple; this breast was once sore when she suffered from mental symptoms for three months. 2 (3).

Great fear of death during paroxysm of pain in heart at night. 7 (7) [1 M].

20. Inclined to be sarcastic and fault-finding. 1. 6 (3).

* Cross and fault-finding, could not speak a pleasant word to any one. 8.

Hysteria in evening, laughing and crying, jumping up and lying down, but could not stand, fell to right side. 1 (19).

After going to bed could not keep from laughing; this lasted for about half an hour, after which abdomen and feet were very cold. 1 (85).

Felt too lazy to reach out hand for water, while very thirsty. 1 (19).

Dislike to read or think. 6 (3).

HEAD.

Pain about middle of r. lambdoidal suture, through to same point on l. side. 1 (2).

Sharp pain passing from r. temple in front of r. ear to lower part of it. 1 (1,102).

Sharp pain in middle of r. side of head. 1 (3).

Pain over r. parietal bone. 1 (7).

30. Was awoke at night by severe pain over r. eyebrow, passing from outer to inner end, and leaving it very sore. 1 (8).

Pain behind r. ear. 1 (13, 18, 24, 35, 38, 58, 70, 74).

Sharp jumping pains behind r. ear. 1 (381.).

Pain in r. temple. 1 (14, 18, 21, 40, 99).
Pain over r. eye and in front of l. ear. 1 (13).
Pain over r. eye. 1 (14, 22, 25, 28, 29, 36, 37, 44, 45, 55, 61, 68, 76, 84 99, 111, 129, 260, 300).
Pain over r. ear passing up and down. 1 (17.)
Pain in r. side of top of head. 1 (17, 316).
Pain in r. eyebrow. 1 (19, 34, 51, 59, 62, 319).
Pain front of r. ear. 1 (22).
40. Pain in r. side of head. 1 (22, 26, 36, 47, 67).
Very sharp pain in r. side of head. 1 (85, 86).
Pain under r. ear. 1 (31).
Pain all over r. side of forehead. 1 (35, 52).
Pain in r. side of head, passing from front to back. 1 (36).
Pain in r. temple; after it had left, a sensation of cold remained. 1 (38).
Pain in r. side of forehead, about size of a cent; after it ceased, the spot felt very cold. 1 (56).
Pain in r. side of occiput. 1 (58).
Pain over r. eye, passing to top of ear. 1 (52).
Pain behind r. ear, felt cold. 1 (70).
50. Burning like fire, and a thick feeling in a lengthwise strip of two fingers' breadth extending from r. frontal eminence to r. side of vertex, for fifteen minutes. 2 (1 after 3¼ hours; returning next day, and ceasing before noon.)
Pain from the parting of the hair to r. ear. 1 (17).
Sharp pain behind l. ear. 1 (1, 15, 17, 28, 45, 47, 53, 77).
Sharp pain from above outer margin of l. eyebrow to inner canthus of both eyes. 1 (1).
Pain over l. eyebrow. 1 (8).
Extremely sharp pains over l. eye. 1 (353, 361).
Pain in l. side of forehead. 1 (11, 12, 24, 47).
Pain in front of l. ear and over r. eye. 1 (13).
Pain passing from l. ear to l. temple. 1 (13).
60. Pain in l. side of head. 1 (17, 18, 22, 27, 48).
Pain over l. eye. 1 (16, 18, 22, 26, 34, 35, 47, 48, 50, 51, 54, 62, 67, 79, 105, 117, 119, 289, 353, 361).
Dull aching pain over l. supraorbital region; worse from bending forward. 6 (1).
Pain in l. temple. 1 (19, 27, 31).
Pain in front of l. ear. 1 (21, 39).

Pain in l. occiput. 1 (26).
Pain over l. eye, passing from r to l. 1 (36).
Pain in l. side of head passing from front to back. 1 (39).
Pain passing all round l. ear. 1 (39).
Pain under l. ear. 1 (43).
70. L. side of head felt all drawn up. 1 (56).
Pain in l. eyebrow. 1 (66).
Pain passing from front of l. ear deep into brain. 1 (84).
L. temple sore to touch. 1 (74, 75).
Sensation as of pressure on frontal bone at inner canthus of l. eye; felt very sore. 1 (116).
Pain in l. side of head and l. ear. 1 (192).
Pain over l. eye all day. 1 (200).
Pain in l. side of head passing down to shoulder. 1 (220).
On turning head to l. side, a pain passing from l. side of head to r. side of neck, similar to 34th day ; on turning head back again, the pain ceased, and a similar pain came over r. eye ; this occurred several times. 1 (260).
Sharp darting pain on l. side of head from temple to occiput. 6 (1).
80. Pain passing along coronal suture from l. to r. 1 (6, 19)
Pain passing from l. to r. side of head. 1 (34).
Pain passing from above l. ear round in front to r. temple. 1 (7).
Stitch above l. eye a little back of eyebrow ; cannot move the eye without excruciating pain. 2 (5).
Pain in both temples. 1 (42, 384).
Pain in both eyebrows. 1 (82).
Pain in both sides of head. 1 (109).
Dull sick headache in frontal region, after lunch at noon, no other time ; with sensation of something rising from stomach to mouth, no taste to it ; a permanent sensation. 1 (196 to 200).
Nearly every day, a sharp pain over eyes. 1 (59, 72, 253).
Severe headache all day through temples, worse from motion and looking down. 1 (293, 294).
90. ₀Pain in forehead like a tight band ; when walking the brain seems to shake. 5.
Forehead feels very heavy, with a tendency to fall forward. 1 (294).

Sharp pain in forehead, passing back and forth from one temple to the other. 1 (3).

Pain in forehead and both ears. 1 (5).

Frontal region very sore, but not to touch. 1 (8, 100).

Soreness of whole front of head on waking. 1 (11).

Pain in forehead passing from l. to r. 1 (17).

Pain in forehead all over. 1 (21, 22, 27, 37, 41, 77, 290).

Pain all over top of head and forehead. 1 (344).

Pressure of hand on top of head causes pain in both ears and top of forehead. 1 (6).

100. Sharp pain in forehead and all over top of head. 1 (34).

Pain in top of head. 1 (13, 20, 25, 30, 42, 260).

Pain in top of head and r. and l. sides of neck. 1 (19).

Pain across top of head. 1 (26).

Pain in top of head and l. ear. 1 (17, 316).

Pain in the parting of the hair. 1 (25).

Head aches all over top, and feels all drawn up. 1 (111).

°Heavy dull pain, with sensation of heat on top of head, as after being up all night. 5.

°Pain extending from region above ears through ears into muscles of neck. 5.

Pain all over top and back part of head. 1 (18, 22, 29).

110. Dreadful pains behind ears and in occipital region. 1 (299).

Aching pains all over occiput. (1, 59).

Pains all over head. 1 (25, 117).

Little pains shooting through head. 1 (287).

Pains in every part of body, mostly through head. 1(287).

°Neuralgic pain in forehead, embracing region of mirthfulness, rationality, comparison, intuition, suavity; also the same pain sometimes in occiput; pain extending to organ of combativeness, and through whole ear down to muscles of neck; aggravation in the regions described above, by the least draught of cold air, with coldness of the parts. 5.

Vertigo. 1 (53, 122).

Feels very light-headed when head is moved suddenly. 1 (344).

Head feels very light. 1 (100).

Head feels dull. 1 (23).

120 Head feels very heavy and inclines to left. 1 (22).

Head feels all contracted with pain. 1 (12, 34).

Shooting pains all over head and abdomen. 1 (3).
Pain in back of head. 1 (7, 14, 21, 24, 25, 37, 43).
Heavy and confused feeling in head. 6 (1).
Desire to have head high when lying down. 6 (1).
Head feels large, and as though all the blood in the body had gone into the head. 6 (1).
Head feels confused, and as if it were tossing on a rough sea. 6 (2).
Head aches all over ; feels very large. 6 (2).
Head feels worse before rising, 6 (3).

130\. Pain in both temples, principally l., with distention of the veins ; pain throbbing and extending down to front of ear, to upper jaw, but not to teeth. 1 (694).

0 Pain in l. side of head and over both eyes, through l. eye and head to occiput. 5.

0 Drawing in neck-muscles and pain in occiput, feeling cold to the touch ; better from warm applications. 5 [1 M].

Head felt strange, heavy, and dull, with a sensation as though she could not hear, though she could. 3 (5).

Between 1 and 2 p. m. fine thread-like pains passing through head in every direction, accompanied by nausea and loss of appetite. 3 (6).

0 From much fatigue and loss of sleep when nursing a patient, had feeling of sickness at stomach and heat in head ; the heat was objective and subjective, commencing in upper forehead and extending gradually all over head, and followed by tingling down spine, which made her move her back from side to side; during the heat in the head, stomach felt lifted up when she moved. Is subject to these symptoms from over-fatigue, and they then last till she has rest and sleep. One dose of C M (Fincke) relieved in one hour (*without rest or sleep*), and next day she was well. This action of the drug was subsequently verified for the second time on the same patient. 4.

EYES.

Pain through r. eye inwards. 6 (2).
Pain in r. eyeball. 1 (294).
Pain in r. eye, with twitching. 1 (16).
Severe pains in both canthi of r. eye. 1 (19).

140. Pain in inner canthus of r. eye. 1 (56).
Pain in outer canthus of r. eye. 1 (70, 78).
Pain passing from outer canthus of r. eye to a point below eye. 1 (27).
Pain passing from outer canthus of r. eye to r. temple. 1 (74).
Pain from inner canthus of r. eye to end of nose. 1 (2, 40).
Pain from inner canthus of r. eye to corner of mouth. 1 (9).
Severe pain in r. eye, causing lachrymation. 1 (57).
Dryness of eyeball, so that the lid would stick to it as if it wanted lubricating, preventing opening and shutting of eye or winking. 1 (182).
Throbbing in r. eyelid. 1 (338).
Swelling of r. upper lid, which increased to a large stye, the lid and all round eye being swollen and red; on third day it broke in two places and discharged copiously. 1 (74 to 79).
150. Pain in l. eye. 1 (24).
Pain in l. upper eyelid. 1 (273),
Burning pain l. upper eyelid. 1 (352).
Pain in outer canthus of l. eye. 1 (22).
Pain in inner canthus of l. eye. 1 (57).
Pain from inner canthus of l. eye to end of nose. 1 (36).
A little sore spot in inner canthus of l. eye 1 (52).
Water causes eyes to smart. 1 (58).
Washing eyes in cold water causes a sensation as if needles were sticking into them. 1 (113).
160. ^{0} Neuralgic pains in eyes. 5 [10 M].
Eyelids feel swollen. which is not the case. 1 (1).
Can only elevate upper lids half-way. 1 (1).
Looking at a bright light dazzles and makes her close eyes; no pain. 1 (51).
Small white pimples appear above inner canthus of each eye, half-way to brow; no inflammation round them. 5 [1 M].
Sight fails; eyes tire very easily. 7.
^{0} Her sight has improved. 2 (6).

EARS.

Pain in r. ear. 1 (3, 9, 17, 21, 25, 30, 36, 40, 81, 102).
Pain in r. ear and underneath it. 1 (12, 22).

Pain in and behind r. ear. 1 (30).

170. Painfulness of r. external ear (concha), with burning like an ulcer, also when touched. 2 (5 at 4 p. m.)

Pain passing from r. ear to shoulder. 1 (117).

Sharp pain from lower part of r. ear passing down about four inches. 1 (267).

Pain in lower part of r. ear. 1 (279).

Pain from r. ear to lower part of inferior maxillary bone. 1 (17).

Pain in front of r. ear. 1 (42).

Sharp pain in l. ear. 1 (3, 17, 18, 19, 26, 59, 68, 101, 104).

Pain in l. external. 1 (34, 53).

Pain in front of l. ear. 1 (272, 300).

Burning in l. external ear. 1 (52).

180. Pain in l. ear and r. side of head. 1 (17).

Pain in l. ear, and sensation as if there were a gathering. 1 (35).

Sharp pains in front of l. ear, sometimes shooting up to eye, and at other times downwards; continuing all afternoon and evening. 1 (278).

Pain in front of l. ear, and at the same time in l. side of neck. 1 (282).

Aching in both ears. 1 (282).

Shooting pains in and behind ears, and all over face. 1 (286).

Pains in external ears and behind them. 1 (288.)

Sharp pain inside both ears. 1 (1, 5, 15).

Burning of both ears. 1 (24).

190. ⁰ Swelling under l. ear about size of hazelnut, attended with great soreness; at the same time mouth kept filling with saliva; similar lump appeared two days afterwards under r. ear, and the flow of saliva increased so as to cause nausea; the swelling of parotids continued several weeks. 8.

⁰ Reverberation of voice when speaking. 5.

Buzzing sound in r. ear. 1 (40).

Sensation as if she could not hear, but she could.

Nose.

Pain in r. side of nose. (170).

Pain in l. side of nose. 1 (42, 77).

Pain in end of nose. 1 (37).

Itching of nose inside and outside. 1 (23).
Itching of nose inside. 1 (52).
Itching of end of nose. 1 (31).
Nose felt sore when touched. 1 (122).
200. Ridge of nose extremely sore ; it feels sore to touch or or from the least movement of facial muscles; the l. side is the worst and somewhat swollen. 1 (398 to 403).
Coryza. 2 (3).
Catarrh of r. nostril. 1 (70).
Catarrh of r. nostril only in morning ; the discharge smelt sour. 1 (57).
Catarrh of l. nostril. 1 (48, 49).

FACE.

Pain passing from corner of mouth to forepart of r. axilla. 1 (1).
Pain along r. inferior maxillary bone. 1 (14, 24, 25).
Pain in r. side of face. 1 (25).
Pain passing from r. ear to under chin, and then up to l. ear. 1 (47).
Pain passing from middle of l. cheek to near corner of mouth. 1 (1).
210. Pain passing from behind l. ear to middle of chin. 1 (1),
Pain in lower part of l. cheek. 1 (10).
Pain in l. side of face. 1 (18, 25).
Pain in front of l. ear passing up and down. 1 (12).
Pain under l. ear. 1 (43).
Pain all round lower part of chin. 1 (2).
Pain under lower jaw. 1 (3).
Face feels as if there were one large pain that covered the whole of it. 1 (3).
Pain in and under chin. 1 (19, 21).
Sensation as if lower jaw were dislocated ; motion of jaw caused a creaking sound. 1 (19).
220. Burning in cheek bones, towards temples and lower jaw. 2 A (1).
Pain all over face, then centering in r. ear. 1 (3).
[0] Darting shooting pain, centered in about middle of r. cheek, extending thence up to eye, especially to r. inner canthus, to ear, and up into right temple ; most severe at centre of cheek, considerably

decreasing the further it extends from centre. 9 [200].

[0] Swelling of face, with pain in head extending down neck and back to feet. 5 [C M].

Wretched appearance, sad expression of face; eyes look as from weeping, though she has not wept. 2 (2).

Great pallor of face, with dark places under eyes. 1 (321, 354).

Great pallor round mouth. 1 (28).

Lips very white. 1 (28)

Great pallor of face. 1 (36, 49 54, 57, 110, 269).

Very dark below eyes. 1 (61).

230. Dark brown circles round eyes, most marked beneath them. 1 (34, 36, 39, 82).

Corners of mouth smart and burn. 6 (1, 2).

Symphysis menti smarts. 6 (2).

Mouth.

Sore on l. side of tongue. 1 (9).

Tongue coated yellow on each side, but none on middle or edges. 1)22, 23).

Tongue coated white. 1 (30, 53).

Tongue coated yellow. 1 (31, 43, 74, 86).

Lips feel very sore and raw. 1 (55).

Lips dry, with great thirst. 1 (24).

Lips very white. 1 (28).

240. Putrid taste in mouth. 1 (52).

Putrid taste in mouth after eating. 1 (60, 61).

Fine spicy taste in mouth. 2 (2).

Taste in mouth like fresh nuts. 2 [30].

Thick bitter mucus in mouth during morning; food tastes fresh, as if there were no salt in it. 1 (111).

Burning in whole mouth, with heat as from drinking whiskey. 2 (2 at 10 a. m.).

Roof of mouth sore. 1 (64).

[0] Expectoration of phlegm or ropy slimy saliva from mouth and fauces. 8.

[0] Sensation of coolness, as of ice in mouth and throat. 8.

Soreness like blisters in mouth and on tongue.

THROAT.

Sensation when swallowing as of a fish bone in throat. 1 (22).

250. Soreness in upper anterior part of throat when swallowing· 1. (22).

Throat feels sore when swallowing. 1 (25).

Spasmodic stricture in æsophagus. 1 (58).

Globus hystericus after lunch at noon, with dull sick headache. 1 (192).

Throat very sensitive to external pressure; the least pressure causes a feeling as if she were choking. 1 (312, 313, 315).

Expectoration of sweet and somewhat viscid mucus, all through the proving; she had had this symptom for years, but some time before the proving had been entirely cured of it by *Stannum* 10 M. 1 (41).

APPETITE.

Hungry all the time; eating does not allay it (this was general through the proving); hunger comes on about 11 am.; has to eat a large quantity before it seems to reach the right spot. 1 (54).

*Desire for dainties. 2 [30].

When first getting out of bed, feels faint for something te eat. 1 (356).

Appetite variable; craving for sweets. 7.

260. Much thirst. 7.

Great thirst; wanted large quantities of very cold water. 1 (19).

STOMACH.

Slight nausea. 1 (28).

Nausea all day, but hunger the same. 1 (54, 62).

Nausea all the morning, 1 (55, 64).

Nausea all day, unaffected by eating. 1 (60).

Nausea all day and evening. 1 (62).

Nausea for smothing to eat, but eating did not relieve it. 1 (342).

Nausea like sea-sickness. 6 (2).

Nausea does not affect appetite. 1 (60).

270. Dyspepsia after eating hot pie-crust. 1 (169).

Pressure in stomach as if she had eaten something indigestible. Heartburn, with sweet taste coming from stomach, without waterbrash. 2 (2).

Great distress in stomach after eating, soon passing up into chest. 1 (400.)

Smelling of *Camphor* caused severe cramp pains in stomach and bowels ; previous to the proving had smelt *Camphor* without the least effect. 1 (26),

ABDOMEN AND HYPOCHONDRIA.

Pain in r. lower part of abdomen. 1 (45, 394).

Feeling as if ulcerated anteriorly over r. short-ribs, worse from touch and when stooping ; slight swelling there ; also all next day till towards evening. 2 (3, 4).

Pain in r. side of abdomen. 1 (77, 384).

Pain in r. hypochondrium. 1 (20, 30, 32, 35, 42, 51, 260, 282, 285, 321, 350).

Pain in a spot just above r. ilium. 1 (17).

280. Pain in anterior superior spine of r. ilium. 1 (24).

Pain from anterior superior spine of r. ilium passing to r. breast. 1 (35).

Pain in front of r. ilium. 1 (43).

Pain in r. ilium. 1 (121, 131).

Pain from crest of ilium passing to inner part of r. thigh. 1 (18).

Pain in l. side of abdomen produced by walking. 1 (51, 69).

Pain in region of l. ninth rib. 1 (6, 259).

Sore pain in l. hypochondrium, relieved by pressure. 7.

Pain from crest of l. ilium to l. breast. 1 (5, 35, 85, 485).

Pain from middle of crest of l. ilium to axilla. 1 (6, 23).

290. Pain in middle of crest of l. ilium passing to anterior superior spine. 1 (10).

Pain over middle of l. ilium. 1 (15, 22, 27).

Pain passing from a few inches above l. ilium to axilla. 1 (23).

Pain in l. hypochondrium. 1 (18, 39, 46, 66, 77, 84; 89 99, 259, 269, 291, 299, 341, 361, 362).

Pain from anterior superior spine of l. ilium passing to l. breast. 1 (32).

Pain about length of finger above l. hip, which would come when leaning back ; lasted two days, followed by severe pain in forhead. 1 (32).

Sharp pain passing across bowels just above navel. and all round body. 1 (1).

*Inflammation and soreness of lower half of navel, passing off by morning, with greenish yellow discharge staining the clothes. 1 (10).

Pain at navel. 1 (12, 34, 52, 58).

Pain above navel. 1 (18, 24, 42).

300. Cramp pains just above navel. 1 (36).

Eating a banana caused a dull zigzag pain to pass slowly from navel downward. 1 (37, 38).

Pain all round navel. 4 (43).

Pain passing across abdomen above navel from r. to l. 1 (10).

Pain passing above navel from l. to r., and then back again. 1 (121).

Pain passing across lower abdomen. 1 (1),

Lower part of abdomen and pelvis feel sore to touch. 1 (7).

At noon, very severe pains in lower abdomen, making her feel sick all over. 1 (256, 257, 258).

Pain in lower part of abdomen in the morning. 1 (282).

Pain along lower part of Poupart's ligament from above down. 1 (17).

310. Sensation of extreme cold passing in a fine line from centre of pubes to a point two or three inches above. 1 (15).

Pain all through pelvis. 1 (23).

Shooting pains in pelvis. 1 (36).

Little short pains all over abdomen, chest, and back, shooting in every direction. 1 (1).

Pains all across abdomen and pelvis, making it almost impossible to stand erect. 1 (5).

Pain all day in abdomen and pelvis, worse on l. side ; not affected by menstrual flow. 1 (32).

Severe pains in abdomen and pelvis during menses, entirely relieved during a sail on salt-water, but returning when she came home. 1 (33).

Abdomen sore and sensitive to touch. 1 (23.).

Abdomen sore to touch, painful from the jar caused by walking. 1 (64).

Pain in bowels. 1 (105, 109).

320. Woke in night with severe pain in bowels. 1 (108).

Cramp in bowels, caused by walking. 1 (37).

Dreadful cramps in bowels as if diarrhœa were coming on, but no stool. 1 (353).

Great distention of abdomen after eating. 1 (64).

Pain from crest of ilium, either side, to sacrum. 1 (2).

Pain passing from middle of crest of each ilium to centre of dorsal region. 1 (27).

Pain all round waist and hip. 1 (114).

Pain all round waist. 1 (119).

Pain commencing at waist and passing to top of r. breast. 1 (337).

RECTUM AND STOOL.

Severe pain passing through abdomen during stool; felt very sore inside. 1 (82)

330. Stool preceded by shooting pains across abdomen, which are relieved by stool. 1 (2, 18).

Before stool, pains in breasts and upper abdomen. 1 (45, 457).

Pain in abdomen before stool. 1 (18, 25, 26).

Before stool, the hands exhaled a fæcal odour, which passed away after stool. 1 (52 to 60).

The first intimation of a stool is a terrible fæcal odour from the whole body, relieved by stool. 1 (286).

Hands exhale a fæcal odour generally in morning and before stool, relieved by stool. 1 (52, 53, 54, 60).

After stool, pain in l. side of abdomen, chest, and heart. 1 (123).

After stool, feeling of exhaustion relieved. 1 (19).

Urgent inclination to stool; felt as though there were a great ball in rectum, much straining, and some flatulence, but no stool and no relief from the flatulence. 7 (8) [1 M[.

Frequent ineffectual urging to stool. 1 (21, 106, 107).

340. Frequent desire for stool, with tenesmus. 1 (106).

Urgent desire for stool, but can pass nothing, only sit and strain. 1 (282).

Great tenesmus, no constipation, stools are quite soft. 1 (21, 28).

Straining at stool causes pricking pains in thighs passing from middle front down to knees. 1 (39, 40).

At night, as soon as she undresses, urgent, but always ineffectual desire for stool. 7.

Great dread of stool. 7 (5).

Slight constipation. 1 (11).

* Constipation. 1 (288).

Constipation, no stool ; these days the hands exhaled a fæcal odour. 1 (53, 54).

Diarrhœa; when at stool, pain passing from anus to tip of coccyx, and also in lower abdomen. 1 (140)

350. Watery diarrhœa all the morning, with pain in abdomen. 1 (49).

Stools smell like rotton eggs. 1 (362).

Great soreness round anus extending three inches up rectum inside. 7 (1).

Constant pressure and soreness at anus, waking her at night. 7 (1).

Soreness round anus. 1 (8, 14, 16, 34, 53).

Anus sore ; the contact of urine with it causes intense pain. 1 (15).

Anus swollen and sore. 1 (59).

Throbbing and beating in rectum and glutei muscles. 7 (1).

Creeping, itching, and crawling round anus, extending three inches inside rectum, relieved for a short time by rubbing. 7 (7).

Shooting pains in the rectum. 1 (19).

URINE.

360. Urination followed by a thick yellow discharge. 1 (3).

Soreness of urethra during urination. 1 (19).

Pain in urethra during urination. 1 (23).

Very severe pain in r. side of abdomen before urination, and sometimes, but not often, lasting during urination, ceasing with it. 1 (209).

⁰ Intense burning of vulvæ internally when urinating. 5.

⁰ Burning and scalding of the parts when urinating. 5.

Constant and urgent inclination to urinate, with cutting pain streaking up urethra after each passage. 7 (2).

Constant and urgent desire to urinate, passing only a few drops at a time, 1 (9).

Frequent and urgent desire to urinate, but can pass only a little. 1 (260).

Urgent desire to urinate, increased by urination. 1 (380 to 420).

370. * Frequent and violent urging to urinate, with passage of a large quantity each time. 1 (240).

* Urine causes intense pain when coming in contact with the labia, which are very sensitive. 1 (2).

Sound of running water produced urination ; no power to restrain it. 1 (2),

* Urinates very frequently large quantities. 1 (28, 105, 106, 107, 109, 115).

Profuse urination when first rising. 1 (120).

Frequent urination, passing large quantities of pale urine. 1 (260).

Urinating when coughing or walking across the room.

Passed a great quantity of urine and frequently. 1 (240).

⁰ Involuntary urination in large quantities several times during night. 8.

⁰ Delay of urination for some time, though the desire and opportunity occur. 5.

Urine stains a dark yellow. 1 (3).

380. ⁰ Urine dark brown, bad-smelling ; no sediment, but cloudy as *Camphor* before a storm. 8.

Shooting pains in urethra and retum. 1 (19).

FEMALE SEXUAL ORGANS.

Menses commenced to-day, very cold hands. 1 (4).

Menses commenced with considerable pain in lower abdomen ; blood bright-red. 1 (4).

Pain across abdomen during menses. 1 (7).

Two or three days before menses feels tired to death. 1 (393).

Menses commenced normal in character and quantity. 1 (32).

Menses commenced, normal in every respect, but too early ; no pain. 1 (57).

Menses commenced too early. 1 (82).

Menses commenced too early; no pain. 1 (108).

390. Menses very dark. 1 (58).

Menses black and thick. 1 (192).

Menses almost black. 1 (5, 7).

° Menses too scanty and often too late. 9.

Leucorrhœa on first rising in morning; none during day or night. 1 (19, 69, 72, 120).

Profuse greenish-yellow leucorrhœa. 7 (2).

Profuse creamy yellow leucorrhœa. 7 (7).

Leucorrhœa white. 1 (182).

Leucorrhœa all day. 1 (122).

Leucorrhœa all day, worse in morning. 1 (123).

400. At times bloody leucorrhœa. 7.

Pain in region of r. ovary. 1 (1, 61, 62, 70, 72, 83).

° Diseases of r. ovary when there is excessive pain. 8.

Pain in l. ovarian region when lifting anything. 1 (118, 300).

Pain in region of l. ovary. 1 (22, 33, 69),

L. ovarion region very sore and weak. 1 (121).

L. ovarion region very weak and painful when walking. 1 (182).

Pain in both ovarion regions while walking. 1 (64).

Constant pain all day in ovaries and lower abdomen. 1 (82).

Sore pain over uterus, sore to pressure, worse next day. 6 (2, 3).

410. Dragging-down sensation in pelvic region. 6 (2).

° For some degree of uterine prolapsus, but especially when, and only when, they complain of an inability to walk in consequence of excessive fatigue. 10.

* Lobulated growths on each side of vagina, nearly filling it; extremely sore and sensitive to touch, or from the pressure caused by sitting; coming on gradually, and lasting more than three months. 7.

Itching of labia minora, 1 (23).

Itching of labia majora. 7 (56).

* Extreme soreness and rawness of labia and entrance to vagina, with profuse greenish-yellow leucorrhœa. 7 (56).

LARYNX AND CHEST.

Pain in r. hypochondrium when laughing hard, coughing, or going upstairs. 1 (192 to 196).

Sharp pain at top of r. breast. 1 (1, 36).

Sharp pain passing into upper r. breast, about an inch deep; very sore to touch after the pain. 1 (1).

Pain from upper r. breast directly through to back. 1 (1).

420. Pain under r. breast. 1 (17, 18, 19, 27, 43, 53, 61, 102).

Pain in r. side of r. breast. 1 (10, 18, 67, 131).

Pain in r. breast. 1 (19, 25, 52, 67, 286).

Pain over r. breast. 1 (21, 23).

Pain from below r. breast to l. shoulder. 1 (39, 40).

Pain passing into chest under right breast. 1 (68).

Pain from forepart of r. axilla to corner of mouth. 1 (1).

Pain in r. axilla, 1 (8, 19, 32, 35, 45).

Severe pain in r. hypochondrium passing under breasts and up between them, better when leaning to left. 1 (198, 264).

Dreadful pains all the evening under r. breast, extending a little below waist. 1 (304, 305)

430. Constant pain under l. breast, worse when bending forward. 1 (1).

Pain under l. breast. 1 (5, 24, 28, 29, 31, 55, 60, 286).

Pain in l. breast. 1 (7, 28, 31, 33, 37, 44, 76, 81, 341, 357).

Pain in sternal end of l. clavicle. 1 (8).

Pain passing through l. breast from below upward. 1 (14).

Pain in l. axilla. 1 (18, 19, 38, 45, 58, 70).

Pain passing from l. breast four inches below. 1 (19).

Pain in l. side of l. breast. 1 (22, 106, 112).

Pain over l. breast. 1 (24).

Pain in l. hypochondrium passing under l. breast. 1 (27).

440. Pain from l. axilla to waist. 1 (30).

Pain from l. breast to a point in front of anterior spine of l. ilium. 1 (35).

Pain in and below l. breast. 1 (47).

Sudden sharp stitches under l. breast, so that for a moment she could not draw a breath. 1 (192) to 201).

Hard pain back of l. breast. 1 (264, 305, 316).

Painful spot on top of l. breast. 1 (321).

Lancinating pains under l. breast, which took away the breath. 1 (325.

Severe pains under l. breast at every inspiration. 1 (336).

Sensation in region of heart as if a fire were there, with a feeling as if heart would burst, or at times as if a heavy weight were lying on it, all of which spreads from this region over the whole inner and outer chest, 2 (1).

Burning and pressure on heart, with fear and anxiety, similar to the attack yesterday. 2 (2, returning again on 3).

450. Awoke at midnight with severe pains about heart, which seemed as if it had almost stopped beating, with a numb pain about heart, lips, and tongue ; great fear of death ; when the pains passed off they left great soreness round heart ; tingling in lips and tongue ; could not lie on l. side ; felt numb and strange all over ; pulse intermittent. 7 (8) [1 M.]

On waking had a distressed feeling all through chest, and felt as if a deep inspiration would relieve, but it did not. 1 (280).

Little sharp pains passing through chest and back. 1 (337).

Pains starting three inches below breasts and passing up to them. 1 (18).

Pains all over breasts 1 (24, 131).

Pains between breasts. 1 (28, 269).

Pains in and below both breasts. 1 (30).

Pains in both breasts. 1 (42).

Sore spots in both brests. 1 (107)

Severe pains between breasts most of the time. 1 (269).

460. Pain passing from l. to r. axilla. 1 (198).

Pains passing from lower to upper end of sternum and then down again. 1 (1).

Pain from lower end of sternum passing to l. about three inches. 1 (1).

Pain in region of sternum. 1 (21).

Pain in lower end of sternum. 1 (30, 39).

Hot flashes from lower chest passing up to chin. 1 (47).

Pain in upper end of sternum. 1 (59).

A few minutes after taking the dose, the patient felt heaviness, aching, and soreness in lower lobe of l. lung; after ten days, says the pain has left that locality, but has extended up whole of l. side, producing a feeling of great weight and difficulty of taking a full inspiration; on attempting to do so, she said the breath was cut short by a catching pain, and she dared not attempt anything but a short and almost suppressed breath; she was under great depression of spirits, but this may have been caused by the fear of poisoning which she expressed. 8.

⁰ Air-cells expanded after taking the medicine. 8.

⁰ Short respiration and nausea relieved in a case of heart-disease. 8.

470. ⁰ Great shortness of breath; the patient "Can't get his breath." 8 [50 M. and C M].

⁰ Breathing much freer than usual. 3 (1) [10 M].

⁰ Rough, dry, or tearing cough, with tightness of chest; upper middle and lower chest affected. 8.

NECK.

Pain passing up and down along r. side of neck. 1 (12).

Pain in r. side of neck. 1 (22, 28, 61).

Pain in l, side of back of neck. 1 (10, 38).

Pain in l. side of neck. 1 (38).

Pain from back part of neck to top of r. arm. 1 (289).

Pain all round upper back part of neck. 1 (1).

Pain in back of neck. 1 (7, 18, 22, 101, 116).

480. Pain along posterior border of sterno-cleido-mastoideus. 1 (8).

Pain in r. and l. sides of neck. 1 (19, 20).

Hot flashes all over back of neck and shoulders. 1 (42).

Hot flashes round neck and legs. 1 (50).

BACK.

Pain below . scapula. 1 (18, 67, 80).

Pain with soreness at upper vertebral border of r. scapula. 1 (22).

Pain in r. scapula. 1 (24).

Severe pain under r. scapula. 1 (286, 354).

Pain in r. side of back between scapula and sacrum. 1 (21).

Pain passing up and down from tip of coccyx to r. shoulder. 1 (2).

490. Sharp pain passing from near middle of l. scapula down outside of arm to end of middle finger, and sometimes to end of little finger. 1 (1).

Pain below l. scapula. 1 (18, 28).

Pain in l. side of back from scapula to sacrum. 1 (25).

Severe pain under l. scapula. 1 (272, 291).

Pain running up back from waist, l. side. 1 (381).

Constant pain all day in region of l. kidney. 1 (6, 80).

Pain in l. sacral region, worse when taking a long breath. 1 (130).

Bunch as large as a 2-cent piece on l. side of coccyx, with sore pains branching up about eight inches; the bunch rapidly lessened in size, and in two hours was only the size of a small pea, but did not entirely dissappear for forty-eight hours; for two years she continued to have a swelling and pain at coccyx preventing her from sitting with any comfort. 7 (5).

Pain passing from coccyx down r. thigh. 1 (18).

Pain passing from tip of coccyx to r. shoulder, up and down. 1 (2).

500. Pain in coccyx. 1 (14).

When crossing r. leg over l. a sore sensation felt in coccyx. 1 (24, 131).

Slight aching in sacrum. 1 (57, 63).

Very sore sensation (not to touch) at and near sacrum. 1 (25).

Pain in sacrum. 1 (24, 30, 39, 83).

Pains each side of sacrum. 1 (42).

Pain in back from sacrum to scapulæ. 1 (72).

Pain passing up back from sacrum. 1 (19).

Pain in back part of waist, passing from r. to l. 1 (26, 47).

Pain in lumbar region, 1 (12, 52).

510. Pain or aching in small of back, relieved by leaning backward, for three or four days. 1 (220).

Pain passing from lumbar vertebræ to half-way up dorsal, and then shooting off into both scapulæ. 1 (1).

Pain between scapulæ. 1 (2, 28, 38, 43, 45, 51).

Severe pain in back, passing up and down from scapula to coccyx. 1 (37).

Pain from back through to lower end of sternum. 1 (10).

Pain all over back and sides. 1 (22, 27).

Pain all over back, which ached and felt very sore; was better while using red ribbon, but afterwards became worse, the aggravation being caused by an impending storm, which she sensed twelve hours in advance. 1 (24).

Back feels very sore and aches. 1 (26, 53).

Severe zigzag pains passing from r. to l. across middle of back. 1 (26, 47).

Fine crawls. as of water running down back. 2 A (1).

520. Dull ache all over back, and in r. arm; canuot bend body far forward, as it causes intense pain in coccyx; when stooping, as in picking anything from floor, has to incline body to one side or other. 1. (321).

Back aches the whole length of spine. 6 (2).

UPPER EXTREMITIES.

Sharp pain in all the r. fingers except little finger. 1 (1).

Pain in r. last two fingers when using them. 1 (7).

Pain in r. little and ring fingers. 1 (19

Pain in r. little finger. 1 (21. 78).

Pain passing up r. little finger. 1 (27).

Pain in middle joint of r. little finger. 1 (32).

Pain in palmar surface of r. index and middle fingers. 1 (39).

Pain in r. middle finger. 1 (42, 43, 109).

530. Pain in r. thumb. 1 (24, 73).

Itching of r. thumb. 1 (48).

Pain in, palmar surface of r. third fiinger. 1 (51).

Pain in dorsal surface of r. third finger. 1 (58).

Pain in end of r. middle finger. 1 (19)

Pain in r. index finger. 1 (67, 68).

Pain in r. index and middle fingers. 1 (297, 300).

Pain in joints of r. fiingers. 1 (383).

Pain in metacarpal and second joints of r. third finger. 1 (259).

Pain across r. metacarpal-phalangeal joints. 1 (324).

540. Pain in metacarpal-phalangeal joint of r. little finger. 1 (26).

Pain between thumb and inner fingers of r. hand. 1 (61, 88).

Pain between r. first and second metacarpal bones. 1 (14, 18).

Pain in dorsal surface of r. hand. 1 (14, 18, 28, 56).

Pain in palm of r. hand. 1 (18, 40).

Itching in palm of r. hand. 1 (24).

Pains all through r. hand. 1 (26).

Grasping anything with r. hand causes pains to pass from all the fingers into palm of hand. 1 (26).

Violent itching of a liver spot on right hand. 2 A (1).

Pain in palmar surface of r. wrist passing into thumb. 1 (18).

550. Pain passing from tip of r. little finger to elbow. 1 (304).

Pain in r. wrist. 1 (12, 14, 15, 18, 19, 25, 26, 27, 32, 38, 78, 81, 101, 337, 355).

Pain passing from r. wrist to elbow. 1 (80).

Pain from r. wrist to shoulder. 1 (34).

Swelling in r. arm below elbow, sore to touch, and pains when she moves arm in certain directions. 1 (285).

Pain in r. forearm when using r. hand. 1 (7).

Pain in r. elbow. 1 (12, 18, 19, 75, 78).

Pain from r. elbow to end of middle finger. 1 (66).

Pain passing from from r. elbow to top of r. scapula. 1 (1).

Pain from r. elbow to top of sterum. 1 (1).

560. Pain from r. elbow to nape of neck. 1 (2).

Pain from r. elbow halfway down to wrist. 1 (7).

Upper part of r. arm, just below shoulder, aches and feels sore, but not to touch. 1 (286).

Pain in forepart of r. upper arm. 1 (39).

Aching pain in r. arm above elbow. 1 (182).

Pain from top of r. shoulder to nape of neck. 1 (1, 15, 27).

Pain from r. shoulder passing down to waist. 1 (6).

Pain in r. shoulder passing a short distance down back. 1 (24).

Pain in top of r. shoulder passing to back and upper part of neck. 1 (27).

Pain passing from r. shoulder to elbow. 1 (27).

570. Pain in back of r. shoulder. 1 (30, 32, 37).

Pain from r. shoulder to l. breast. 1 (33, 37).

Pain passing from r. to l. shoulder. 1 (38).

Pain on top of r. shoulder. 1 (69).

Rheumatic pains all over r. arm. 1 (320).

Shooting pains from base of l. index finger to end, on dorsal surface. 1 (1).

Pain in l. little finger. 1 (116).

Pain from l. first metacarpal bone to end of little finger. 1 (7).

Pain along ulnar side of l. little finger. 1 (10).

Pain in l. little and ring fingers. 1 (21).

580. Pain in l, middle finger. 1 (28, 78).

Pain in l. ring finger. 1 (29).

Pain in l. thumb. 1 (6, 12, 21, 38).

Rheumatic pains in l. fingers. 1 (260).

Pain in l. palm. 1 (14, 15, 24, 25).

Pain extending from proximal end of l. first metacarpal bone, passing between third and fourth metacarpal bones, coming out on palmar surface, and ending at metacarpal joint of little finger. 1 (7).

Pain in middle of dorsal surface of l. hand. 1 (27).

Pain in l. metacarpal-phalangeal articulations. 1 (45).

Pain in l. wrist. 1 (17, 18, 24, 26, 27, 61, 67, 79, 85, 86).

Pain from l. wrist to middle joint of middle finger. 1 (30).

590. Pain in l. arm just above wrist. 1 (84).

Pain in l. arm passing up between wrist and elbow. 1 (3, 46, 82).

Pain in l. elbow. 1 (22, 28, 38, 44).

Pain in inside of l. elbow. 1 (37).

Pain from l. elbow to back of neck. 1 (6).

Pain in inside of l. arm above elbow. 1 (260).

Pain in l. shoulder. 1 (15, 17, 18, 19, 21, 27, 30, 44, 45, 55. 103, 108).

Pain back of l. shoulder. 1 (36, 100).

Pain from top of l. shoulder to under part of r. breast. 1 (1).

Pain in l. shoulder and side. 1 (73).

600. Pain in top of l. shoulder. 1 (42).

Pains in last two fingers of both hands. 1 (18).

Fingers ached so that she could not use them. 1 (182).

* Skin under nails looks dirty, it cannot be washed or scraped off, for two days. 1 (10, 11)

Pains in both hands passing to ends of fingers. 1 (6).

Pains in hands passing in all directions. 1 (7).
Pains in both wrists, encircling them. 1 (4. 9).
Pain with slight stiffness in both wrists. 1 (10).
Pain passing from wrists to end of fingers, on dorsal surface. 1 (7).
Pain in both elbows. 1 (5).
610. Hot flashes in both arms from wrists to shoulders. 1 (38).
Pains shooting from top of shoulders to middle of dorsal region, uniting and passing down to sacrum. 1 (2).
Pain in front of shoulders. 1 (12).
Pain in both shoulders. 1 (22, 33, 325).
Itching of both shoulders. 1 (31).
Shoulders and hips lame. 1 (118).

LOWER EXTREMITIES.

0 Pain like gout in r. toe, sometimes slight pains upwards in r. limb; toe will not bear contact of any shoe; pain always the same standing, walking, or lying down; continued exercise aggravated it, 9.
Pain in r. little toe. 1 (7).
Pain in top of r. great toe. 1 (316).
Pain in r. great toe. 1 (42, 43, 58).
620. 0 Sharp cramp-like pains under r. great toe, on first stepping on it after rising. 9.
Pain in top of all the r. toes. 1 (57).
Pain in under part of r. toes. 1 (38).
Pain passing from ends of all the r. toes to ankle. 1 (2).
Pain at back part of r. heel, coming on before 9 a. m. and after 3 p. m. 1 (2).
Pain passing along inner margin of r. foot, and then at a right angle up heel. 1 (2).
Pain in top of r. foot. 1 (17).
Pain in under surface of r. foot; worse from walking. 1 (52, 64, 104).
Pain in l. side of r. foot; when walking the pain would pass down into foot and up leg. 1 (267).
Pain in r. ankle. 1 (21, 24, 42, 43, 129, 289).
630. Inside of r. ankle felt sprained; hurt most when stepping on ball of foot. 1 (118).
Pain in r. ankle, so that she could scarcely walk. 1 (4).
Pain in back part of r. ankle passing up. 1 (17).

Pain in l. side of r. ankle, passing over top of foot to end of toes, then halfway up leg on inner side. 1 (3).

Pain in r. instep. 1 (21).

Pain in r. instep when bending foot. (352).

Pain in r. leg below knee. 1 (28).

Pain in middle of r. tibia. 1 (36).

Pain in r. knee. 1 (27, 31, 34, 39, 56, 273).

Pain above r. knee. 1 (45).

640. Pain in top of r. knee. 1 (73, 79, 117, 282, 296).

Pain in top of r. knee, worse when walking. 1 (1, 2, 12 14, 24, 36, 40, 42, 52).

Pain from under part of r. knee to coccyx. 1 (6, 7).

Pain from forepart of r. knee to anterior-superior spine of r. ilium, and passing back to middle of sacrum. 1 (8).

Pain in top of r. knee and back part of r. leg, 1 (16).

Pain in under part of r. knee. 1 (17, 74).

Pain in under part of r. knee passing halfway up thigh. 1 (17).

Pain in r. knee-cap. 1 (114).

Pain starting from middle of r. leg and passing almost to knee. 1 (27).

Aching of r. leg above and below knee. 1 (114).

650. Pain in l. side of r. thigh. 1 (15).

Pain passing down along back part of r. thigh. 1 (19).

Pain in middle forepart of r. thigh. 1 (23).

⁰ Inflammation and awful pain extending down whole trunk of r. sciatic nerve. 8 [C M and MM].

⁰ Pain in inner side of r. thigh and in r. hip, more or less constant; but worse after rising. 9 [200].

Pain in r. hip. 1 (14, 34, 103, 123, 192, 356).

Pain passing through r. hip from front to back, also in the reverse direction. 1 (4).

Pain in back part of r. hip. 1 (44, 111).

Pain in r. side of fold of nates. 1 (1).

Pain in r. gluteal region. 1 (13, 18, 24, 34, 74, 76).

660. Pain in r. side of r. leg. 1 (26).

Pain in l. side of r. leg, and along r. side above knee 1 (11).

Pain in under side of r. leg. 1 (114).

Sharp pain in large joints of l. great toe. 1 (21).

Pain in ball of left great toe. 1 (24, 51).

Pain just above l. heel. 1 (53).
Pain in l. heel, worse from walking. 1 (55, 59).
Pain in hollow of l. foot, only when walking. 1 (324).
Pain in l. sole. 1 (19, 21).
Pain in top of l. foot. 1 (27, 38).
670. Pain passing along middle of l. foot to second toe. 1 (15).
Pain in l. instep and heel, worse from walking. 1 (267).
Pain in l. ankle. 1 (12, 18).
Pain in l. ankle and heel. 1 (60, 61).
Pain passing from inner side of l. ankle to heel. 1 (10).
Pain just below l. knee, on front of leg. 1 (19).
Sharp pain under l. knee passing down back of leg to ankle, and then round ankle. 1 (1).
Pain from top of l. knee to l. lower abdomen. 1 (3).
Pain in l. knee, passing three or four inches up thigh 1 (7).
Pain from inner side of l. knee, passing three or four inches up thigh and then down to heel. 1 (7).
680. Pain in l. knee. 1 (11, 22, 24, 33, 35, 43, 62, 76).
Severe pain in top of l. knee, joint of r. great toe, and outer canthus of r. eye, at the same time. 1 (19).
Pain under l. knee. 1 (21, 29, 75).
Pain in top of l. knee. 1 (29, 42, 51, 53, 78, 81, 108, 115, 192).
Pain in l. knee passing to ankle. 1 (45).
Pain passing from top of l. knee and then running up again. 1 (273).
Pain passing from under part of l. knee and short distance up thigh. 1 (27).
Sharp pain starting from middle of l. leg and passing up over knee. 1 (25).
Severe pain in top part of l. leg below knee. 1 (35).
Painful spot near upper part of l. leg in front. 1 (14).
690. L. thigh very sore to touch. 1 (358).
Pain in l. hip. 1 (14, 78, 107, 119).
Pain in lower part of l. gluteus maximus. 1 (46).
Throbbing in outside of l. leg. 1 (35).
Balls of feet covered with little corns, which are very painful when walking. 1 (354).
All her corns become painfully sensitive. 7.
When standing for a long time, feels as if her knees would give way. 1 (273).

Pains in both knees. 1 (31).
Pain in top of knees. 1 (18, 113).
A great many pains in legs from knees down, for a few days. 1 (225).
700. A spot just above knee is very sore to touch. 1 (78, 256).
Pain in both hips. 1 (23).
Shooting pains passing in all directions round hips. 1 (85.)
Lameness in both hips. 1 (315).
Pain in both gluteal muscles. 1 (21).
Gluteal muscles feel very sore from the jar caused by walking. 1 (43, 45).
Soreness of gluteal muscles on pressure. 7 (7).
⁰ Pains in thighs and hips. 9.
Soreness in streaks, extending from anus down back of legs to heels ; can feel a rigidity (not raised) where the soreness is. 7 (2).
The sore rigidities almost gone, but succeeded by a crawling as if maggots were creeping up to anus, for two days. 7 (6, 7).
710. Hot flashes in lower limbs. 1 (47).

FEVER.

Great coldness as if a chill were coming on ; hands, particularly the fingers, and feet, particularly the toes, icy cold ; could not keep warm in bed covered with clothes, and during day sat near a stove, but could not get warm. 3 (2).
During evening chilliness attended with weakness of back, as though she would not be able to walk, yet she could walk with an effort. 3 (4).
All day felt an agreeable sense of coolness through body ; this passed off, and she then felt a warmth throughout abdomen. 3 (3).
Hot flashes inside body pressing from below upward. 1 (38).
Strange restlessness at night, feeling of great heat all over, the body covered with a light perspiration, just enough to feel uncomfortable. 3 (1).
Slight perspiration during sleep between 4 and 5 a.m. 3 (7).

SLEEP.

Continual yawning all day. 1 ((1, 22, 24).

Dreams, with fear of falling. 1 (15).

Cannot recall her dreams. 2 (20).

720. Dreams often of dead persons, of little children who are born and die; that brothers who really still live are dead or have died. 2 (22).

Dreams fatiguing dreams all night. 6 (2).

Awoke with the impression that she had dreamed of dreadful pains in chest; does not know whether it was a dream or a reality. 1 (290).

Dreams of cattle. 6 (2).

Dreams that rare beefsteak, of which she is very fond, made her sick; the following morning, on attempting to eat beefsteak, she became nauseated, and did not get over it for some hours. 1 (650).

Could not fall asleep before midnight. 2 (1).

Sleeplessness after midnight. 2 (20).

Wakes for several mornings at 4 a. m. precisely; subsequently wakes at 5 a. m., for several mornings. 1 (16).

Very restless several nights, waking frequently with pains in abdomen and chest, and tossing about, and throwing off the covering. 1 (37).

Desires to lie down, but has no wish to remain after doing so. 1 (37).

730. Slept at short intervals; sleep did not refresh her. 3 (4).

Very sleepy all day. 1 (28).

Does not feel sleepy, but has a strong desire to go to bed. 6 (1).

Cannot sleep on r. side. 1 (269).

Cannot go to sleep without putting arms over head. 1 (394).

*Impossible to lie straight in bed, finds herself continually lying diagonally across bed. 1 (525).

Cannot sleep straight in bed, must be crosswise; when she wakes, no matter in what position she was when she went to sleep, she finds herself across the bed. 7.

Has to lie on l. side, as she is comfortable in no other position. 7.

SKIN.

Very restless at night from itching all over body as soon as she is covered in bed. 1 (94, 95).

Itching of both shoulders. 7, 1 (31).

GENERALITIES.

740. Sensitive in almost every portion of body, especially the feet, as if little pieces of flesh were being cut or pinched out; the pain is so severe and sudden that it makes her start from her seat; succeeded by a stinging sensation, which soon passes off, leaving no soreness. 7.

⁰ Excessively cold neuralgic pain in cartilages of ears, worse in r., with tingling as if frost-bitten; rubbing with difficulty restored warmth; pain in forehead, occiput, in region above ears extending down through ears into neck muscles, and in eyes: these pains are all lancinating neuralgic, and are all icy-cold, as if produced by an extremely fine ice-cold needle; all worse from the least breath of air; skin sensitive to touch as in inflammatory rheumatism. 5 [1 M].

Small shooting pains all over her in morning. 1 (2).

Body ached and felt very sore when leaning forward. 1 (35).

The pains, with but few exceptions, are all superficial. 1.

Pains passing through body from front to back and from dorsal vertebræ to stomach, causing nausea. 1 (43).

Throbbing in various parts of body. 1 (48).

Ached all over as if from a cold. 1 (118, 273).

A great many pains all over her. 1 (220, 273).

Felt very sore from the pains of the preceding day. 1 (221).

750. Pains all over, but not of any consequence. 1 (281).

Neuralgic pains all over. 1 (289, 290).

⁰ Short flying darting stitches in different parts of the body, quite painful, but bearable, appearing in head, eyes, ears, and face, as well as in extremities, not confined to any especial locality. 9 [200.]

° Great physical exhaustion, caused by overwork, completely relieved. 1 (1) [repeatedly verified by Swan and others].

Except when stated, she has not experienced the slightest fatigue, though working all the time during the proving. 1.

° Anticipated fatigue from a laborious day entirely prevented by 1 M (11).

Felt tired and completely exhausted all day, relieved by stool. 1 (19).

Felt perfectly exhausted, as though she coud not move. 1 (28).

Feeling of weakness in whole body, as after great fright or fear. 2 (20).

Felt lame all over. 1 (290).

760. General malaise, only during evening. 1 (315).

The shooting pains caused complete exhaustion, as if she could not bear another pain, but this soon ceased. 1 (3).

Felt once in a while as if her whole body were asleep. 1 (28).

Felt as if benumbed with cold, though not really cold. 3 (2).

° Could not catch her breath, felt numb and strange all over. 5.

Trembling feeling, as if about to faint ; it lasted till 11 a. m., when I partially swooned. 3 (3).

Trembling of whole body while walking. 6 (3).

The first days the symptons ceased between 9 a. m. and 5 p.m. 1.

The pains during the proving were intensified by a coming storm, the approach of which was felt some twelve hours previously. 1.

Pains were aggravated in damp room or basement, but relieved if there was a fire. 1.

770. All symptons relieved after 4 p.m. 6 (2).

Pains were generally worse morning and evening. 1.

The pains having ceased, were reproduced by placing a blue ribbon on her head. 1 (70).

No symptoms to-day till she placed a bow of yellow ribbon on head, which made her sick all over, followed in a few minutes by severe pains across upper abdomen. 1 (71).

During the proving, the pains could be stopped by placing a red ribbon on head and another on neck in front. 1.

Very restless all evening. 1 (21).

Cannot bear to have any clothes over her at night ; felt cold without any, but even the sheet seemed to be too much. 1 (82).

° Could not lie on left side. 5.

Desire to lie down. 6 (2).

Desire to sit with feet high. 6 (3).

780. Desire to lie down, but do not wish to remain after doing so. 6 (2).

Wasted, haggard, and wan. 7.

Before fainting, great heat and burning in abdomen. 3 (2).

After exercising in warm weather or in hot room, would frequently faint ; after fainting, very weak, particularly in ankles, being almost unable to walk. 3 (2).

Felt better all day than I had for years. 3 (3).

Prostration from mental exitement. Rushmore.

FRAGMENTARY PROVING.

(*Trifolia Pratense*—Mrs. B. After CM.)

SLEEP.

Entire sleeplessness all night, without restlessness or desire to sleep. As refreshed in the morning as if she had slept sound. (Coff. test.)

Unrefreshing sleep during menses.

MENTAL.

Exceedingly low spirited ; everything looks dark and discouraging.

EYES.

Suffusion of eyes, causing obscuration of light.

Is myopic. Since taking the drug finds eyesight improving.

While reading, from one page to the next, a dark flash occurs in the left eye.

Fine white substance gathers on the tarsal edge of the lower lid; it washes off with difficulty, leaving a redness at roots of the lashes.

HEAD.

Headache every afternoon in frontal region; relieved by pressing both temples.

Just before headache commences, feels exceedingly tired.

STOMACH.

Nausea after food has been down five or ten minutes.

Nausea with menses.

Vomiting food twice after eating.

ABDOMEN.

The usual quantity of flatus in lower intestines, greatly diminished.

ANUS AND RECTUM.

Piles exceedingly sore came on during menses, protruding like a bag on right side to front of anus.

MENSES.

Menses delayed a week.

Painless.

Very tired during menstrual period.

UPPER EXTREMITIES.

Soreness as if bruised, or like a touch of rheumatism in upper part of left Brachialis anticus.

LOWER EXTREMITIES.

Painful sensation of Gluteus Medius at its junction with the upper edge of left ilium.

On the posterior side of left thigh, from nates to knee, aching as soon as she lies down at night; movement and flexing the leg relieves. Only at night.

Fatigue in the legs, do not feel it when sitting. When standing. and especially walking, it is exceedingly apparent. Seems impossible to put one foot before the other.

LAC CANINUM (Dogs Milk).

ARRANGED BY E. W. BERRIDGE, M. D.

The sign 0 signifies a merely cured symptom. The sign * signifies a pathogenetic symptom also verified by a cure : if placed anywhere besides the beginning of the symptom, it signifies that the portion of the symptom to which it is attached, from stop to stop, has been thus verified. R. signifies right, and L. left. The unbracketed figures following a symptom denote the authority ; those in round brackets denote the day on which the symptom occurred, the day being reckoned from the first dose, or from the first of any potency where that potency is mentioned.

All of Lac Caninum were from 30th and upwards.

The names of corresponding remedies in italics are, with a few exceptions, kindly added by Dr. Ad. Lippe.

PROVERS NAMES.

1. Laura Morgan, M. D.
2. G. K. Hazlitt, (from Thos. Wildes, M.D.)
3. Miss W. (from ditto.)
4. Mr. J. L. H. (from ditto.)
5. H. K., a woman ; (from S. H. Talcott, M. D.)
6. Mrs. M. A. Wheelwright, (from Sam'l Swan M. D.)
7. Wm. White, M. D.
8. Geo. D. Gale, M. D.
9. De Forest Hunt, M. D.
10. E. C. Chase, M. D.
11. Geo. D. Grant, M. D.
12. Samuel Swan, M. D.
13. Ad. Lippe, M. D.
14. C. Lippe, M. D.
15. E. W. Berridge, M. D.
16. A. K. Hills, M. D.
17. W. E. Payne, M. D.
18. A. Reisig, M. D.
19. W. C. Pardee, M. D.
20. C. F. Nichols, M. D.
21. Jos. Finch, M. D.
22. Thos. Wildes, M. D.
23. W. P. Wesselhoeft, M. D.
24. B. L. B. Bayliss, M. D.
25. D. A. Hiller, M. D.
26. G. H. Carr, M. D.
27. J. C. Boardman, M. D.
28. C. G. Schlick, M. D.
29. Sarah J. White, M. D.
30. H. W. Taylor, M. D.
31. S. Mills, Fowler, M. D.
32. J. A. Biegler, M. D.
33. W. Eggert, M. D.
34. J. R. Haynes, M. D.
35. E. A Farrington, M. D.
36. G. C. Brown, M. D.
37. J. C. Guernsey, M. D.
38. Mr. A. (from G. G. Gale, M. D.
39. Mr. B. (from ditto)
40. Mrs. Taylor, (from H. W. Taylor, M. D.
41. Miss Grace Taylor, (from ditto)
42. Baby Taylor, (from ditto)
43. A lady (from E. A. Farrington, M. D.)
44. Mr. N. (from C. Lippe, M. D.
45. J. C. Morgan, M. D.
46. C. Pearson, M. D.
47. — Sullivan, M. D.
48. D. Dever, M. D.
50. J. E. Winans, M. D.
51. John F. Miller, M. D.
52. C. W. Butler, M. D.
53. Miss Clara Gardiner, (from E. W. Berridge, M. D.)

54. Mr. Fryer, (from ditto)
55. A lady (from W. Eggert, M. D.)
56. A lady patient, (from L. Morgan, M. D.)
57. Count Ghererdo Freschi.
58. Paz Alvarez, M. D.
59. Miss Lizzie Moore, (from S. Swan, M. D.)
60. Several patients (from S. J. White, M. D.)
61. Several patients (from D. A. Hiller, M. D.)
62. Arthur Deliven, (from E. B. Nash, M. D.
63. Miss Nell, (from ditto)
64. H. N. Guernsey, M. D.
65. E. A. Ballard, M. D.
66. Arabella Kennedy, M. D.
67. Mrs. Baxendale.
68. G. W. Sherbino, M. D.
69. C. Carleton Smith, M. D.
70. Mrs. Anderson.
71. Mrs. Burdick.
72. Patient of Dr. Nichols.
73. W. S. Gee, M. D.

RECORD OF PROVERS.

1. Laura Morgan, M. D., æt. 24, being in sound vigorous health, took three doses of 32nd centesimal on March 13th, 1871, six doses March 14th, and nine doses March 15th. On May 17th symptoms ceased, returning May 25th. (Symptoms after 32nd potency are marked 1a.) On 27th she took one dose of 1m (Fincke, marked 1b,) and on 28th a dose of 40m (Fincke, marked 1c,) in evening; the symptoms which followed abating on June 19th. On June 21st, she took a dose of 75m (Fincke, marked 1d.) Symptoms ceased, with menses, on July 20th, and on 28th and 30th she took one dose, each day, of CM (Fincke, marked 1c.) From these doses symptoms continued, usually at menses, till January, 1873, and then ceased. On January 23d, 1873, for "an oppression and sense of suffocation in chest," similar to what she had experienced on 6th day of proving, she took one dose of 10m (Fincke, marked 1d,) which relieved the oppression and was followed by some very marked and characteristic symptoms. There was a renewal of many of these symptoms for several months at menses.

2. G. K. Hazlitt, æt. 43; health generally good, sometimes has rheumatism, fair complexion, clear pale skin, sandy hair, blue eyes, nervo-sanguine temperament; commenced proving 200th (Swan,) September 28th, 1876; no medicine after 11th day. (Swan's potencies were prepared from Reisig's 17th).

3. Miss W., æt. 27; subject to slight catarrh of head, occasional sick headache, weak bowels, diarrhœa every summer, never had leucorrhœa or any uterine trouble, menses regular and painless, except occasional pain on vertex on last day; menses always four or five days, bright red, drying dark, wash out easily; commenced proving 200th (Swan,) September 16th, 1876, during menses; afterwards took 1m (Swan marked 3a).
4. Mr. J. L. H., æt. 28; fair complexion, clear skin, light hair, temperament prettily evenly balanced; grandparents lived to from 80 to 85; parents always healthy; one paternal aunt died of phthisis, and a brother of diphtheria; has always had good, though not robust health; subject to slight catarrh of the head, and an occasional slight involuntary movement of eybrows: commenced proving 200th (Swan,) September 16th, 1876; afterwards took 1m (Swan, marked 4a).
5. H. K., proved 200th (Swan).
6. Mrs. M. A. Wheelwright, took two globules of 200th (Swan) daily for two weeks.
7. Wm. White, M. D., commenced proving 200th (Swan,) October 24th, 1876.
11. G. D. Grant, M. D., proved 50m (Swan).
12. S. Swan. M. D., took two doses CM (Swan).
30. H. W. Taylor, M. D., proved 200th (Swan).
38. Mr. A. æt. 16; nervous temperament, had chorea from fright when young, mother rheumatic; proved Cm (Swan) November, 1879.
39. Mr. B. æt. 19, dark complexion; proved Cm (Swan) November, 1879.
40. Mrs. Taylor, wife of H. W. Taylor, M.D., æt. 41, brunette, above average heighth, full figure, weight 140 lbs., strong, health excellent, nursing a baby six months old. August 31st, 1878, took six doses of 200th (Swan). September 1st, ditto; September 2nd, about 12 doses; first symptoms appeared next night. All symptoms subsided by about September 8th. In previous winter had malignant diphtheria, with the same symptoms except the hypergastric pain and palmar itching.
41. Miss Grace Taylor, æt. 7, fair, tall, slender, bony; had membraneous diphtheretic croup when a year old, leaving enlarged tonsils and cervical glands. Had

diphtheria the previous winter. Took 15 to 20 doses September 2d and 3d 1878; symptoms commenced September 3rd, ceasing by September 7th. (200th potency of Swan).

42. Baby Taylor, six months old, a fat, white boy, with black eyes and hair, had symptoms from the medicine absorbed through his mother's milk.

43. A lady æt. 25, in excellent health, but had never menstruated, took four doses of 10m (Swan,) daily for three or four weeks. Symptoms commenced October 19th, 1878. How soon after first dose is not stated; in the schema, Oct. 19th is called the first day. The symptoms without a date, occured between November 8th and January 5th.

44. Mr. N., æt. 22; proved 31st centesimal. Three years ago had chancre on glans, removed by external applications, and Mercury internally. Since this suppression, has suffered from excessive mental depression, and has at no time since the chancre, felt any of the bouyancy of youth, there is a want of ability to concentrate his mind on his studies; he has an indolent, painless enlargement of the lymphatics, principally of the neck and submaxillary regions. Since the proving his mental and general condition is much improved. Took first dose on night of November 25th, 1878, before retiring; Nov. 26th, a dose at 9 a. m. continuing it every four hours; last dose at night, November 28th.

53. Miss Gardiner, took one dose of CM (Fincke,) December, 1882, for nervous affection of throat. Afterwards took a dose of CM (Fincke) morning and evening, for six doses, beginning April 24th, for sick headache (marked 53 A); afterwards took MM (Fincke) thrice daily for fourteen days, for throat trouble, in August, 1883 (marked 53b).

54. Mr. Fryer, æt. 76, suffering from urinary weakness, took a daily dose of CM (Fincke,) for seven days, beginning May 13th, 1881.

55. A lady twice took 50m, with the same result each time.

56. A lady took 75m and suffered an intense aggravation of her symptoms.

59. Miss Lizzie Moore, took CM for sore throat until relieved. (Swan's patient.)

60. Several patients took potencies for relief of their symptoms.

61. Symptoms noticed "in all cases where from 1M to CM have been given to patients."

62. Arthur Deliven, æt. 25, spare, light complexion, dark hair and eyes, commenced taking 200th (Boericke and Tafel), evening October 26th, 1883; took six No. 30 pills every hour through 27th; omitted it afternoon of 28th; commenced again morning of 29th, when the first symptoms appeared. Took no medicine through the night at all.

63. Miss Nell, æt. 32; blue eyes, light brown hair, bilious temperament; commenced to take Lac. Can. 200th, Oct. 30th, 1883; took No. 30 pills, six every hour. Stopped proving November 8th. First symptoms appeared Nov. 2d.

66. Dr. Arabella Kennedy, æt. 24; dissolved two globules of Lac.Can.CM (Fincke,) in water, and took a teaspoonful every hour. Had symptoms almost immediately after first dose, but no more, though she continued the medicine.

67. Mrs. Baxendale, æt. 29; took a dose of Lac. Can. CM (Fincke,) twice a day for fourteen days, for dysmenorrhea which it decidedly relieved, but produced toothache very soon after commencing the medicine. Has has had the same kind of pain in face and teeth from over-fatigue or much worry, but never at stated hour, or lasting so many hours at a time, or so many days in succession.

70. Mrs. Anderson, suffering from diphtheria, took 3d dec. from a chemist, with much relief; after the improvement set in, a new symptom appeared, drinks returning by the nose.

71. Mrs. Burdick, took DMM (Swan,) under Dr. Swan's direction.

72. A patient of Dr. Nichols took DM (Swan), three weeks after diphtheria.

PUBLISHED LITERATURE.

N. A. J. H. IV. (n. s.) 251. Organon, II., 204, 238–9, 281, 311–2, 341, 484, 509; I., 364; III., 27, 102–3, 338, 379, 362, 522; IV., 130. H. M. X., 213, 279. H. P. I., 350, II., 98; III., 218; IV., 64–5, 103, 193, 297–8; V., 388. VI., 21–28. M. A., June, Aug., 1877; Feb., Dec., 1878; Aug., 1879; Oct., 1885 (v. 15, p. 213) v. 18 67 (copied from Organon), v. 17, p. 555–565. U. S. M. I., Jan. 15, 1881, p. 97.

H. W., XVIII., p. 297, 359, 367.

I. H. A. Proceedings, I., 115, 259, 286, 296–7.

H. P., VI., 410–11; VII., 65, 67.

M. A., XVIII., 251.

MIND AND DISPOSITION.

Sensation, or delusion, as if surrounded by myriads of snakes, some running like lighthing up and down inside of skin; some that are in R. side feel long and thin; fears to put her feet on the floor lest she should tread on them, and make them squirm and wind round her legs; is afraid to look behind her for fear she will see snakes there; does not dream of them, and is seldom troubled with them after dark. 1 (38).

On going to bed was afraid to close her eyes, for fear that a large snake, the size of her arm, would hit her in the face; it seemed by the side of the bed, and had its head near hers. 1.

Sensation as if she were going *deranged (*Calc.*) 1.

When she sits still and thinks, she sometimes has the most horrible sights (not always snakes) presented to her mental vision; she is terribly afraid that they will take objective form and show themselves to her natural eye; and she sits and looks under the chairs, table, sofa, and everything in the room, expecting, yet dreading to see some terrible monster creep forth, and feeling all the time that if it does it will drive her raving mad (*Hyos.*). She is not afraid in the dark; it is only in the light when she imagines that she can see them. Sometimes she feels as if she could not refrain from crying out with terror. 1.

Was afraid for many nights to go to bed, for just before bed-time, a huge snake would coil itself at the side of the bed on the floor, and when she would get into bed, would crawl in too, and get under her. Would much rather have sat in her chair all night, but did not dare to let such powers have control over her; though she never at any time saw the snakes, yet their color, size and movements were always known to her. 1 (38 to 45).

Wake at night with a sensation that she was lying on a large snake. 1c. (172).

After menses, imagines all sorts of things about snakes. 1c. (226).

Woke at daylight, feeling she was a loathsome horrible mass of disease disgusting to herself and to every-one else; could not bear to look at any portion of her body, not even her hands, as it intensified the feeling of disgust and horror. Could not bear to have any one part of her body touch another; *had to keep even her fingers apart from each other; felt if she could not get out of her body in some way, she would soon become crazy; could not think of anything but her own condition. In a short time she fell into a light slumber, from which she woke free from all mental but not physical symptoms. 1a. (38.)

⁰Feels weak, and nerves so thoroughly out of order, that she cannot bear one finger to touch the other. ⁰Nervous throat affection. 15.

Is impressed with the idea that all she says is a *lie; that all her symptoms are unreal, and the result of a diseased imagination; it seems to be very difficult to speak the truth, but continually distrusts things; when reading anything she rapidly changes the meaning, omitting or adding things. 1c. (245).

10. Every time a symptom appears she feels very confident that it is not attributable to the medicine, but is some settled disease. 1c. (38).

⁰Imagines that he wears someone else's nose. ⁰Diphtheria. 20.

Felt very short in morning while walking. 1a. (3)· ditto in evening. (2.)

Finds it very difficult to read understandingly anything requiring a mental effort to follow it. (*Calc.*). 1.

*Very restless; cannot concentrate her thoughts or mind to read; wants to leave everything as soon as it is commenced. (*Nux. Sil. Sulp.*) 1a. (37.)

*Cannot collect her thoughts; confused feeling, causing inability to record symptoms, or write a letter. 1. (*Lach.*) 3d., (18 after 1M).

*When speaking, substitutes the name of the object seen for that which is thought. (*Amm.c. Calc. Sep., Sulp.*) 1. (Jan., 1873).

Cannot speak correctly half the time. (*Calc., Chin., Graph., Hep., Lach., Lyc.. Nat.c., Nat.m., Nux., Sep.*) 1.

Cannot remember even a short paragraph after reading it, but can remember other things; it seems to affect only what she has read. (*Lach., Nat.m., Staph.*)

Very *forgetful; in writing, uses too many words or not the right ones; very *nervous. (*Bov., Graph., Hep., Lach., Lyc., Nat.c., Nat.m., Nux., Sep.*)

20. Tendency to omit the *final letter in a word; writing also only the last letter in words of two letters, and having to go over her writing to make corrections before sending it. (*Lach., Nux.m.*) 1.

Very *absent-minded; makes purchases and walks off without them. (*Agnus, Alum, Anacard, Caust, Nat.m., Sep.*) 4 (6).

Very *absent-minded; went to post a letter, bought and affixed the stamp, and then brought the letter home in her hand. (*Con. Dulc. Lach., Nat.m.* 3 (7).

°Cannot bear to be left alone for an instant. °Diphtheria. 14.

Came into my office crying, fearing she was contracting consumption. (*Calc., Paullin, Sep.*) 35.

°Fears she will become unable to perform her duties. °Nervous throat affection. 15.

°Fits of weeping two or three times a day. Parenchymatous metritis. 32 (CM).

Depression of *spirits; *doubts her ability; doubts of her success in her profession; thinks she will have heart disease and die of it (*Lach.*); thinks she is of no importance in life. 1c (128).

°Gloomy feelings increased as headache gets worse. °Parenchymatous metritis. 32 (Cm).

30. *Chronic "blue" condition; everything seems so dark that it can grow no darker. (*Lyc. puls.*) 1.

°She is very "blue"; felt hopeless and quite discouraged. °Diphtheria. 37.

*Despondent and hopeless: believes her disease incurable, and that it is not the effect of the drug; does not care whether she lives or dies. (*Act.*, *Bry.*, *Calc.*, *Lach.*) 1.

*Feels as though she had not a friend in the world, and could cry at any moment; there seems to be nothing in the world worth living for; would like to die any time. (*Aur.*, *Lach.*, *Sep.*) 1a (37).

°Thinks she is looked down upon by everyone, and feels insulted thereat. 26.

Anxiousness. 4 (10).

°No desire to live. 22.

Feeling of great mental anxiety. 53 (1)

Great fear of falling down stairs at times. (*Borax.*) 1.

°Very nervous; constant dread; a feeling she was going to become unconscious. °Diphtheria. 51.

40. During night, very restless; waking often frightened, and not knowing where she was. °Diphtheria. 51.

°Fear of death, with anxious expression of countenance. °Diphtheria. 9.

On lying down, either by day or night, she begins to think how terrible it would be if a very sharp pain like a knife should go through her, and the thought of it causes great mental distress; she always imagines that the pains are these that would pass through the body. 1e. (128.)

°Easily excited. °Parenchymatous metritis. 32 (CM).

°Too excited to allow any further examination of throat. Diphtheria. 25 (CM).

°Very easily startled. Parenchymatous metritis. 32.

*Nervous and irritable. 2 (11).

Extremely irritable when not in sopor. 20 (CM).

*Very cross and irritable while the headache lasted, (*Nux.*) (21, 23.)

°Child cries and screams all the time, especially at night, and will not be pacified in any way. 26.

50. °Attacks of rage, cursing and swearing at the slightest provocation. 26.

°Cursing and swearing. 26.

°Swears like a pirate at every little thing. 26.

*Intense ugliness and hatefulness in all moods and tenses, past, present, and future. 1e. (209 to 216).

Writes to her best friends all sorts of mean and contemptible things. 1c (208.)

In afternoon, solemn and serious mood; not inclined to jest or talk, though at other times could do so with pleasure. 8a (2).

Exalted feeling of sensorium. (*Plat.*) 2 (8).

*Cross and irritable. 1a (22, 24.)

°Wakes distressed, and obliged to rise and occupy herself in some manner; fears she would be crazy. °Parenchymatous metritis. 32.

°Exceedingly nervous. °Parenchymatous metritis. 32.

60. °When awake, very irritable and cries constantly. 26.

°When the paroxysms of intense nervousness come on, feels like tearing off her clothes; would take off her rings; could not bear anything to touch her, especially over L. ovarian region, from which she frequently lifts the bed-clothes. °Ovaralgia. 68.

°After inhaling the gas for extraction of teeth, very strange sensation in head (such as he felt when going off under the gas); sometimes imagines the heart or breathing were going to stop, or otherwise frightens himself, and this makes heart beat violently; occasionally very depressed, and fancies he is going out his mind. 15.

Worries herself lest the pimples which appear on thighs during menses will prove to be little snakes, and twine and twist around each other. (See legs.) 1e (172).

°Omits the final letter or letters of a word, when writing; mentions, in speaking, the object seen, instead of the object thought of. 15.

HEAD.

Sharp lancinating pain, extremely fine, passing in a zigzag line from R. side of forehead to an indefinite point in occiput; the pain is instantaneous, and is sometimes repeated; as soon as it is felt, she lays aside whatever she is doing and lies down, from an indefinite dread that it will return; if at night, she goes to bed at once; has great dread of the pain, though it is not very severe; it recurred for several days afterwards. 1c (174.)

Sharp throbbing pain in r. side of forehead; then in l. side of forehead slightly. 4a (39).

Headache only in afternoon, extending from r. temple to r. malar bone. 1a (33, 37.)

Sharp pain in r. temple and through forehead. 4a (16).

Sharp darting pain in r. temple, then across forehead, lasting only a minute. 4a (22).

Sharp pungent pain in r. temple, and then dull pain in forehead. 4a (44).

Sharp pain like a stab in r. temple, at 7 p. m. (*Alum.*, *Bell.*, *Canth.*, *Cycl.*, *Meny.*, *Phos.*, *Phos.ac.*, *Rhus.*, *Sars.*, *Strout*, *Verb.*) 2 (8).

Neuralgic pain in r. temple and through temples and forehead, all the afternoon. 4 (2).

Throbbing pain just above r. temple, then sharp pain in socket of r. eye and in r. temple, disappearing quickly. 4a (6) after 1m.

At 8.15 p. m., sharp throbbing pain in r. temple. 4 (3).

Pain in petrous portion of temporal bone, down neck on r. side. 1b (after taking *Ramex*). April, 1873.

Dull pain through r. side of head. 4a (45).

Fine lancinating pain in r. side of head. 1 (Jan. 1873).

Headache on r. side of forehead. 1a (34, 36).

*Pain in forehead during afternoon, first on l. side, then on r. 1a (18).

Headache over l. eye on first waking, and great pain in pelvis, most marked at r. ovary. 1a (18).

80 Headache *over l. eye, on first waking. 1a (18).

Steady aching pain in l. eyebrow, several afternoons, relieved by keeping head steady. 1e 286.

Acute pain in forehead over l. eye. (*Act.*) 4a (8).

Pain in l. temple, passing from it to l. ear, and then to molar teeth of left upper jaw. 1a (24).

At 10.45 a. m., darting pain in l. temple, alternating to r., then both together ; of short duration. (*Puls.*) 4 (1).

Very severe sharp cutting pains in l. temple, waking her at night several times. 3a (17).

Pain in l. side of head and l. temple, very severe from 11 a. p. to 3 p. m. 3a (17).

Headache quite sharp, extending back over l. side of head. 2 (8).

Neuralgic pain in l. side of head, followed by a film over l. eye, with inclination to rub it off ; rubbing does not relieve. 1f. (*Spig.*) August, 1873.

Headache first on one side of forehead, then on the other. 1a (13).

90. Headache in upper forehead. 1c (5).

Slight frontal headache on waking. 1a (62).

*Frontal headache. 1a (7, 17); 1c (3).

*Pain in forehead almost all day. 1c (12).

Slight frontal headache. 1a (54, 55) ; 1a (7).

*On going into the cold wind, felt a terrible pain in forehead as if it would split open, relieved on going into warm room. 1e (*Aur.*. *Nux.*, *Rhus.*) (172).

Headache in upper part of forehead, with sensation of a broad band pressed firmly across forehead from one temple to the other. 1a (*Coca*) (2 to 5, 7, 9, 10, 12).

Pain in centre of forehead, worse on rising after stooping. 8a (2).

Slight dull pain across forehead, all forenoon. 4 (6).

Occasional slight dull pain across forehead, with stitches during last three days. 4 (14).

100. Dullness across forehead, and stitches.

Slight pain across forehead. 4a (29).

At 8 a. m., sharp transient pain across forehead, succeeded by dull heavy feeling across forehead and temples.

At 11.45 a. m., sharp darting pain across forehead, disappearing quickly. 4 (53).

Pain in forehead, darting back over l. ear, and slight darting pain across forehead. 2 (1).

Darting pain across forehead and over eyes. 2 (2).
Darting pain from forehead over r. eye. 2 (3).
Headache over l. eye in forenoon. 2 (5).
Headache across forehead. 2, (6).
Headache over both eyes, extending back over l. ear. (2, 7).
110. Occasional sharp pains in forehead. 2 (8).
Darting pains through forehead, dull pains over eyes. (*Puls.*) 2 (12).
Sharp throbbings pains in front part of head, especially over l. eye, (*Act.*, *Kali.*, *Nux.m.*, *Spig.*, *Verat.*, disappearing after a two hours sleep. (*Phos.*, *Puls.*, *Mix.*) 3 (9).
Acute pain across over eyes and bridge of nose. 43 (19).
⁰After midnight, very severe frontal headache, and a piercing pain on vertex; pain was immediately removed, and she slept calmly for some four hours, and in the morning was much refreshed and altogether better. ⁰Typhoid pneumonia. 25 (40m).
⁰Pains and throbbing in temples. ⁰Dyspepsia. 25 (10m).
*Headaches are always in upper and forepart of head, however different in character. 1.
⁰Arose in morning with heavy dull frontal headache; about 9 a. m., a severe sharp pain on vertex, apparently coming from nape (*Silica*,) then stretching across the head forward; pain is so severe that he presses vertex with his hands; neck stiff; bending head forward, or lying down causes congestion, increasing the pain; then again the pains will subside for a short time and begin anew, either in front part of head, or nape, or all over head at once; when the pain is frontal, it causes lachrymation. 25 (40m).
From 6.15 p. m. to 7.15 p. m. pressure on vertex. 3. (46).
Slight pressure on vertex. 3. (51).
120 Slight pressure on vertex and over eyes, the day before menses ceased (*Calc.*). 3. (54).
Much heaviness in vertex, with complete loss of appetite. 44. (7).
Dull pain in r. temple and r. eye, with pressure on vertex during menses. 4a (16).
Stiffness and lame feeling in occiput on turning head, with soreness on pressure. 7 (2).

°Beating in occiput. °Parenchymatous metritis. 32 (CM).

°Darting pains from occiput to forehead. °Parenchymatous metritis. 32 (CM).

°Occipital headache, with shooting pains extending to forehead. 36.

°Aching and pain in occiput. °Parenchymatous metritis. 32 (CM).

Headache nearly all day. 1a (65).

130 Slight headache. 1a (30).

Slight headache for a short time. 1a (28).

Slight headache on first waking. 1a (63, 64).

*Severe headache. 2 (2, 4). °Diphtheria. 12.

Severe headache on rising at 7 a. m. 2 (3).

°Severe pressure on brain. Parenchymatous metritis. 32.

*Headache. 1a (25 to 27, 5, 8, 10, 24, 15, 16, 22). Diphtheria. (51, 12, 17, 21).

Bad headache, violent, too bad to work. 2 (11).

*Headache in afternoon, principally over l. eye (*Acon. Kalm.*). 2 (4).

*Headache worse by noise or talking, better by keeping quiet; confused feeling in head (*Calc.c.*) 3a (18).

Intense headache, entirely relieved by cold water application, but soon returned, not however as severe, (*Arsen.*, *Bell.*, *Bry.*, *Cycl.*, *Glon.*, *Zinc.*) 1a (6).

140 °Headache from below eyes over whole head and top of shoulder. °Parenchymatous metritis. 32 (CM).

Headache and nausea on waking, lasting all morning, (*Kalib.*, *Nux.*) 1a (11).

Head feels heavy, dull, and stupid, as though it would be impossible to make the least mental effort. (*Bell,*) 1a (37).

Dull headache, at times quite sharp and cutting. 2 (10).

In afternoon felt headache coming on, which became much worse about an hour after going to bed. 39 (2).

*Pains in head during day, first on one side then on the other; it seems perfectly unbearable; relieved on first going into the air, but soon grows worse. 1a (21).

°Headaches seem unbearable, and are attended by pain in lumbar region; all pains cease as soon as throat gets worse. °Diphtheria. 20.

Menses commence slight; second and third days very free; fourth day less free; ceasing on fifth day; during menses, slight pain in lower abdomen, very low down; dull pain in r. eye and temple, changing next day to l. side and temple; pressure in head; nausea; the headache and nausea aggravated by motion, relieved by quiet. 3a (15).

°Head aches, mostly through temples, darting, stabbing; sometimes begin on r. side, and sometimes on l.; always going from one side to the other. 26.

Head aches all over, worse over r. eye, worse by spells; rolls head from side to side, with great distress, with pains in bones of head. °Diphtheria. 12.

150 °Frequently wakes with sick headache, which seems to commence at nape. °Nervous throat affection. 15.

Sensation as if brain were alternately contracted and relaxed, several times rapidly; generally only when lying down; at various times all through proving. 1 (*Calc. Medorrhin*).

Confused feeling in head, with headache. 3 (18).

At 11.30 a. m. sensation of confusion and pressure through temples and entire forehead, followed by a sensation as if forehead were compressed by a band. (*Apis. Sulp.*) 4 (1).

In afternoon, much confusion of head, making thought irksome. 44 (3).

Stupid condition of head. 44 (11).

In evening some dizziness when walking. 14 (5).

150 *Dizzy sensation with slight nausea. 4a (24).

Weak feeling in head, feeling as if a headache were coming on. (*Ambr. Iod., Phos., Stram., Thuj.*) 3a (19).

°After inhaling diphtheritic breath, is light headed, with tingling on vertex, and slight sore throat; always acts as prophylactic. 25.

160. Constant noise in head, very confusing; worse at night, and much worse at menses. °Parenchymatous metritis. 32 (CM).

°Wakes at night with sensation as if the bed were in motion; noise in head bad beyond description; first thought on waking that the head-board was swaying, and so occasioning the distress, but found it arose from internal causes. ⁰Parenchymatous metritus. 32.

Excessive dandruff on head for past week. (*Alum, Arsen, Lach., Mez., Oleand., Thus.*) 4 (14).

Sore pimples on scalp, which discharge and form a scab ; they are extremely painful when touched, or on combing the hair. (*Mez.*) 1c (209, 214).

Head very sore, and itches almost all the time, worse at night. 1c (209 to 216.)

Slight roughness of the skin of forehead, as of numerous pimples. 4 (4).

Headache from r. temple to r. malar bone. 1a (37).

Headache on l. side of forehead on first waking, soon passing off. 1a (20).

Pain on l. side of forehead on first waking. 1a (21).

Headache first on one side, then on the other. 1a (14).

170. Frontal headache, with the sensation of a band across forehead, 1a (3).

Headache ; band across forehead. 1a (4, 12).

Pain in l. occiputal region running up when moving head. 62 (5).

When she rose to walk across store was very dizzy ; head felt dizzy all the time, but was greatly aggrated when moving ; (has had similiar attacks before) 63 (4).

⁰Sick headaches, begining in nape ; the pain settling gradually in r. or l. forehead. 15.

⁰Headache over eyes, worse when sewing. Pharyngitis. (12).

⁰Headache, both frontal and occipital, aggravated by turning eyeballs upwards. 23.

EYES.

Sharp pain in socket back of r. eye, followed by tenderness in r. temple; both transient. (*Bell.*,) 4a (1m).

Darting intense pain round l. eye (*Spig.*,) 4 (45).

⁰Heaviness of l. upper eyelid, with pain above l. eye. ⁰Rheumatism. 25 (75 m).

180 ⁰Burning in l. eye. ⁰Rheumatism. 25 (75 m).

⁰Agglutination of l. eylids. Rheumatism. 25 (75 m).

Eyes slightly swollen ; profuse lachrymation ; with catarrh. 3 (4).

Eyes swollen and running water. 6.

⁰Eyes watery and discharging. ⁰Diphtheria 22 (CM).

Looking at different objects causes eyes to ache (*Calc.*,) 1d (9 to 11) (after 75 m).

Pain in both eyeballs. 1d (16) (after 75 m).

Pain in eyeballs when looking upwards. 1a (22, 23).

Aching pain in eyeballs. 1c (7, 8,) after 40m.

Pricking sensation in eyeballs; eyes sensitive to cold air. (*Phos.*) 3 (44).

190. *Upper lids very heavy, can scarcely keep eyes open; very sleepy. (*Bell.*, *Caust.*, *Nat. c.*, *Sep.*) 1a (2).

⁰Non-œdematous swelling of upper and lower lids; pink color of lower lids most noticeable on r. ⁰Diphtheria. 14 (30 and 900).

Eyes feel weak during menses. 3 (51).

⁰Dark brown areola under eyes. 26. ⁰Retarded, painful menses. 12.

⁰Eyes dull and lustreless. ⁰Diphtheria. 46.

⁰Heavy pain in eyeballs, with outward pressure. 50.

Eyes twitch, with increase of former nervous symptoms.. 53 (1).

⁰Eyes blurred. ⁰Parenchymatous metritis. 32.

Pain in eyes when reading; followed by a *film over them, apparently requiring to be wiped off before she can see. (*Puls.*) 1c (112).

Film over l. eye from reading or looking closely at anything. 26.

⁰Film over r. eye from reading or looking closely at anything. 1 (26).

200. Nearly all this month, at times, a sensation as if there were something over l. eye, seeming as if it could be removed by rubbing finger over it. The sight is very much obscured; at first she would have it only once or twice a day, afterwards it increased, but now she does not have it very much. 1c (382). (See also under *Head.*)

Difficulty of changing axis of vision. 1d (9 to 11.

Slight inaccuracy of vision. 2 (8).

*Tendency in retina to retain the impression of objects, especially of colors; or somewhat of the object last looked at is projected into the next. (*Nicotin*, *Tuberculin.*) 1e (92).

°Sees faces before her eyes, worse in the dark ; the face that haunts her most is one that she has really seen. 15 (CM).

Cannot read, as it causes pain in eyes ; the letters look as if the light fell unequally upon them, causing some to be very dark, and others to be very bright. 1c (13, 14). (40m.)

Small floating discs before eyes occasionally, and showing primary colors at edge of discs. 1e.

*When reading, the page does not look clear, but seems covered with various pale spots of red, yellow, green, and other colors. 1e (30) after 75m.

°When looking in a mirror by gaslight, after exerting eyes, sees a green spot or a green band before her l. eye, the band slanting downward from l. eye to r. cheek. °Glaucoma. 15. (CM.)

210 °Square or round green spots or brown spots before l. eye, when sun is bright ; sometimes bright spots before l. eye. °Cataract. 15 (CM).

Occasionally, when looking at an object, sees red spots on it (*Hyos.*,) 1d (3).

On going to bed, in dark room, sees many stars, on closing eyes, moving from r. to l. 8a (2).

While looking at an object, appears to see just beyond or out of the axis of vision, an object passing across the field of sight; but on adjusting the eye to see it, is gone; it always appears as a small object, like a *rat or bird, sometimes on the floor, at others in the air. 1c (112).

°Frequent sensation of a film before eyes, with vertigo, and while thus suffering would see a small dark object, like a mouse or bird, coming up to her left. 12 (CM).

°Sees big eyes and creeping things. °Diphtheria. 14 (30 to 900).

°Difficulty in distinguishing objects ; in reading, the letters run together. °After severe diphtheria. (*Nat.*, *Mur.*,) 12 (MM).

°Must have light, yet is intolerent of sunlight. °Diphtheria. (*Acm.*, *Amm.m.*, *Bell.*, *Calc.ac.*, *Calc.*, *Gels.*, *Ruta.*, *Stram.*,) 14 (30 to 900).

°Sensitive to light. °Rheumatism. 25.

Eyeballs feel too large, and as if she must move them about. 53a.

220 Dull aching pain in r. eyeball, accompanied by a feeling of dryness and discomfort, with tendency to lachrymation, l. eye not affected; almost immediately. 66.

(No eye symptoms after 10 m. 1).

EARS.

Pain in r. ear, sometimes intense. (*Bell.*,) 1a (9, 10, 11, 13, 15, 16, 17, 19, 22, 23,). 1c (16).

Pain in r. ear, wrist and patella. 1a (4).

Very sharp pain in r. middle ear, while walking in the wind; had to cover it with hand, which gave entire relief; sharp pain in r. side also. 1f (March, 1873).

Pain in l. ear. 1a (29 to 32).

Pain in both ears. 1a (33).

No pain during day, but is awakened several times during night by sore aching pains in middle and external ear on which she is lying; soon passes off when the pressure is removed. 1f (March 1873).

Dry itching sensation in ear; dry wax. 6.

[0]Green odorless discharge. 12 (CM).

Reverberation of voice, as if speaking in a large empty room; with pain in frontal region, first over one eye and then over the other. 1 (*Caust*). 37.

230. [0]Sounds seem very far off. (*Cann. ind.*, *Cham.*, *Coca.*, *Nitrogen*, *Protox.*, *Nux. m.*, *Petiv*, *Solan. nig.*)

Ringing in r. ear. 1a (24 to 27).

At night, a buzzing in r. ear. 39 (2).

Noises in ears; sensation as though ears were full. 1 (Jan., 1873).

[0]More than any other remedy, relieves deafness from hereditary syphilis. 29.

Pain in r. ear, lasting only a few minutes. 1a (2).

Pain in r. ear for a short time. 1a (3).

Slight pain in r. ear. 1a (4, 21).

Intense pain in r. ear. 1a (14).

Irritation in both ears to throat. 53b.

NOSE.

240. *Sore on r. side of septum of nose ; next day nose sore, constant inclination to pick at it and get the scab off ; nose still sore on 6th day, and on 7th day was very painful to touch ; but on 8th day scab came off nose, leaving it as well as ever. (*Kali bich. Thuj.*) 1a (37).

R. side of nose seems stopped up. (*Sticta, Teucr.*) 1a (37).

Sore spot came suddenly in l. side of nose, high up ; on touching it, it bled very freely ; during afternoon, nose felt as if all filled up, producing a constant inclination to blow it, yet there was not the least discharge. 1c (July, 1872).

L. nostril first dry, afterwards discharging a thin ichorous fluid, *excoriating the nostrils. 40 (6).

Soreness from nose through into throat. 43 (19).

Itching at end of nose; inside and out. (*Cina.*) 1.

Severe cold, followed by swelling and eruption of lips and throat. 3 (May, 1873.)

Feels as if she had taken cold in head, stuffed feeling in nose and throat. 3 (2).

Stinging feeling in nose at 7.15 p. m., with occasional sneezing during day. 3 (3)

Very bad cold in head, sneezing and occasional cough, eyes slightly swollen, fluent coryza, profuse lachrymation ; better next day. 3 (4).

250. Watery discharge, followed by dry sensation in nose. 6.

*Constant discharge of thin watery fluid, which slightly excoriates edges of nostrils. (*Nit. Acid,*) 1a (5).

*Coryza ; constant watery discharge from nose, excoriating nostrils and upper lips. 1a (37). *Arum tri.*

°Nasal discharge, excoriating nostrils and upper lip. °Diphtheria. 14.

°Excoriating mucous discharge from nostrils. °Diphtheria. 9.

°Coryza, with discharge of thick white mucous. 14.

*Fluent catarrh from both nostrils, with sensation of fulness in upper part of nose. 1a (5).

Catarrh of nose, with bloody discharge ; some of it falls into throat. (*Nit. ac.*) 1c (209 to 216).

⁰Profuse nocturnal nasal discharge, like gonorrhœa, staining pillow greenish yellow. (*Merc.*, *Puls.*) 12, 26.

Cannot clear head, nose stuffed. 43, (19).

260. *Head so stuffed she can hardly breathe. 3 (8). *Lyc.*, *Nit. ac.*, *Nux.*)

*Stuffed feeling in head, sensation as of a severe cold in head. 3 (2, 5).

⁰One side of nose stuffed up, the other free and discharging thin mucous at times and thin blood; these conditions alternate, first one nostril stopped up and the other fluent, and vice versa. ⁰Diphtheria. 14 (30 and 900.)

*Considerable sneezing. 1a (5). (*Gels.*, *Verat.*)

⁰Epistaxis when speaking or swallowing. ⁰Diphtheria. 20.

⁰Copious epistaxis at 4 p. m., returning at intervals. ⁰Diphtheria. 23.

Bad smell in nose. 1e (35, 36.) (*Aurum.*)

Cannot bear smell of flowers; (*Graph.*, *Lyc.*) they seem to send a chill over her. 6.

⁰Fluids escape through nose while drinking. ⁰Diphtheria. 9, 20, (CMM.) 22, (CM.) 24, 26, 37. (*Bell.*, *Lach.*, *Merc.*, *Petr.*)

⁰Feels as if fluids swallowed would return through nose, but they do not. ⁰Diphtheria. 23.

270. ⁰Nose cold. ⁰Diphtheria. 12.

⁰All drinks return by the nose, nothing being swallowed. ⁰Diphtheria. 37.

Catarrh of both nostrils. 1a (4).

Drinks return by the nose. 70.

*Nose discharges much thin watery mucous. 63 (10).

⁰Two very angry gatherings, one under l. side of nose, and one on upper l. nostril; both came to a head, and discharged matter and blood, and afterwards scabbed over; before the discharge there was shooting pain there. ⁰Sick headache. 15.

Disposition to sneeze, and symptoms of cold in head. 53b.

⁰Nose became so bad that there was fear of destruction of the bones; bloody pus was discharged several times daily; the nasal bones were sore on pressure. 32.

FACE.

R. cheek burns like fire, and is red after coming in from the cold. 43.

°Red circular spot below r. malar bone, burning to touch. °Dyspepsia. 25.

280 Burning of l. side of face, for about an hour (*Asaf.*, *Murex.*, *Nat. m. ol. an.*, *Phos. ac.*, *Spig.*,) 1a (4).

°Flushes on l. cheek. °Dyspepsia. 25.

Pain as from knife-thrust from under l. zygoma up to vertex. 71 (15 minutes) 12 DMM.)

°Anxious expression of countenance. °Diptheria. 9, 22, 23, 51.

°Cheeks red. °Diphtheria. 23.

°Face flushed. °Diphtheria. 10.

°Face burns, feels dry. °Diphtheria. 20.

°Face flushed, swollen and hot. Diphtheria. 25.

*Burning flushing of face. 6.

Face very red for one hour after rising, then pale, followed by natural color again. 3 (11).

290 *Marked pallor of face. 3a (2).

Orange red spots on face and hands, appearing and dissappearing suddenly ; small in size, circular in shape, not elevated, nor having any sensation. 1a (3).

°Countenance pale and care-worn. °Diphtheria. 46.

°Face very red, and then suddenly pale. 26.

°Seems to affect lower lip most, and blisters and fever sores on lips are amenable to its influence. 26.

Pulsation of superior coronary artery in upper lip, simulating something living in it. 1f (Sept., 1873).

*Lips dry and peeling off. (*Arum tri*, *Nat. m.*) 3 (15).

Lips parched and burn. 3 (17).

*Lips dry and parched, but mouth constantly full of frothy saliva. 1 (b).

Lips very dry, but no thirst. 1a (18).

Lips burn and feel very red, (*Arum tri.*) color of face natural. 3 (13).

300. °Jaw cracks while eating. °Dyspepsia. 25.

On secon day of menses, face flushed and hot ; in two hours afterwards face became cool and of a yellowish pallor. 3 (2).

Lips, throat and tongue parched and dry, on third day of menses. 3 (27).

*Face flushed. 62 (5.)

⁰Face indicates great anxiety. ⁰Diphtheria. 51.

⁰In morning, left superior maxillary feels sore ; most of of the time there is dull pain, worse by exertion ; sometimes throbbing pain, burning, throbbing, aching heat, sensation of fullness ; cannot wear her false teeth from the soreness and swelling of maxillary ; an exacerbation of pain leaves face very sore ; pains better by warm applications, but only cold applications relieve the soreness ; wakes about 2 a. m., and does not go to sleep again ; during this time is very restless, face very painful, and life indeed becomes a reality ; thoughts, acts, and sights of the near past, appear before her like a panorama ; feels better when mind is occupied ; cheerful company causes her to forget the pain, solitude depresses her. (*Epulis.*) 65.

TEETH.

Pain in l. upper molars, coming from l. temple through l. ear. 1a (24.) See *Head*, there given fully.

Teeth sensitive to cold water. (*Arg. m.*, *Bry.*, *Calc.*, *Mang.*, *Merc.*, *Nux.*, *Nux.m.*, *Puls.*, *Rhus.*, *Staph.*, *thuj.*) 1a) 22, 23).

⁰Gums swollen, ulcerated, retracted, bleeding, teeth loose; caused by defective nutrition and exposure. (*Iod.*, *Kali.*, *Lyc.*, *Merc.*, *Nat.m.*, *Phos.*, *Staph.*, *Zinc.*) 19, 26.

⁰Paroxysmal gnawing pain in l. upper canine, temporarily yields to any cold application. ⁰Sick headache. 15.

310. Tooth-ache ; the pain used to come on quite suddenly at about 10.30 every night; if not before she went to bed, it would begin almost immediately on lying down or getting warm in bed; so that she was obliged to jump up and often walk about the room ; the pain seemed to begin in a very much decayed r. lower double tooth, but after a while all the teeth on the r. side would ache; it was relieved by the application of cold water or a dose of *Cham.*, which

would often quiet it immediately; it continued for quite a month, coming on each night, and the teeth after feel tender and as if they were too long or too large still; it was often daylight before she could get any sleep at all; the pain was not very bad, it was a dull gnawing sensation, as of a worm gnawing at the teeth, just enough to keep her wide awake; it came on at the same time whether she had her last meal early or late or went without it; if she went to bed earlier and fell asleep, it would wake her up when the hour arrived. 67. (*Syph.*)

MOUTH.

*Tongue coated brown. (*Arsen.*, *Nux.*, *Rhus.*, *Sulp.*) 1a (9).

°Tongue generally red and moist. °Diphtheria. 9.

Tongue very red, and coated white. 1a (2, 3).

Tongue pale red, coated white. (*Glau.*) 1a (34).

*Tongue furred whitish at edges, centre and root darker. (*Bell.*) 2 (1).

*Tongue coated, dirty looking, centre to root. 2 (2)

*Tongue coated whitish, except edges, which are red. 2 (3).

°Tongue thinly coated with a dirty white. 27.

°Tongue dirty-coated, yellowish white, and slimy. °Diphtheria. 21.

320. °Slight yellow coating on tongue. Diphtheria. 9.

Tongue coated all over. 2 (4).

Tongue coated all over; less coated in afternoon, edges red. 2 (5, 6).

Tongue dirty, *deeply coated near back and centre, except on edges, *which are bright red; at 9 p. m. tongue looks patched. 2 (9, 10).

Tongue dirty, particularly in centre. 2 (11, 12.

°Tongue dry; and thickly coated grayish-white. °Diphtheria. 25.

Tongue coated *whitish-gray, having an underlying bluish look. 41 (3).

°Tongue heavily coated, and dry to the tip. °Diphtheria. 46.

°Tongue fairly loaded down with a thick coating, yellowish at centre, paler at edges. °Diphtheria. 37.

°Tongue heavily coated white, except a stripe of deep red on edges. θDiphtheria. 12.

330. Tongue relaxed, flabby, with whitish coating. θAcute rheumatism. 52.

Soreness on r. side of tongue. 7 (3).

*Putrid *taste in mouth. 1a (3, 8, 13).

Taste of lead in mouth in afternoon. 38 (2).

°Putrid taste in mouth. θDiphtheria. 9.

Swelling of l. sublingual gland, ranula. (*Calc.*, *Merc.*, *Thuj.*) 1d (20).

Mouth and throat covered with aphthous yellowish-white ulcerations, easily bleeding. 26.

°Stomatitis; stomacace; cancrum oris; nursing sore mouth. 26.

Mouth and throat covered with dark yellow spots. (*Lach.*, *Lyc.*) 1a (37).

Sore on lower jaw, behind r. molar tooth, almost well next day. 1a (8).

340. Folds of inner lining of l. cheek creased and painful. (*Petrol.*) 1.

Roof of mouth very sore, with blisters that break and leave loose skin; any seasoned food causes great pain. 1a (Dec., 1872).

Inside of lower lip feels tender and sore, and looks very red. (*Arum tri.*) 3a (1).

*Mouth very dry. (*Ang.*, *Bry.*, *Lob.*, *Nat.m.*, *Nux.m.*) 6.

°Mouth dry without thirst. (*Nux mos.*) θDiphtheria. 20.

°Mouth dry and parched; drinks little and often. θDiphtheria. 20.

*Increase in quantity of saliva, which is slightly viscid. 1a (2).

*Profuse saliva, saturating pillow. 6.

*During sleep, saliva ran from mouth, so as to wet pillow. (*Merc.*, *Nit.ac.*, *Rhus.*) 6.

Mouth constantly full of mucous, but a constant* inclination to swallow, which *causes pain. (*Apis.*, *Arum tri.*, *Dig. Euph.*, *Hell.*, *Hep.*, *Lach.*, *Merc.*, *Sep.*, *Stram.*, *Sulp.*, *Verat.*) 1a (12).

350. *Frothy mucous in mouth, increased by going into open air, and *after eating. 1a (4).

Mouth full of frothy *mucous; constant inclination to swallow. 1c (1).

Mouth constantly full of slightly viscid mucous. 1a (18).

°Peculiar rattle in mouth, right along tongue; on attempting to hawk her mouth clear, the mucous rattled along tongue quickly and continually; utterance was so indistinct as to be unintelligible, and every word she tried to speak was accompanied by this quick and continuous rattle along the tongue. ⁰Diphtheria. 37.

°Profuse secretion of saliva, sometimes frothy. ⁰Diphtheria. 9.

°Constant salivation and drooling. ⁰Diphtheria. 9, 26.

°Drooling from mouth. ⁰Diphtheria. 22, 26.

°Constant drooling, very profuse, making chin and breast sore. 19.

°Constant spitting and drooling. ⁰Diphtheria. 20, 26.

°Difficulty in articulating, owing to a semi-paretic state of tongue, causing stuttering if she talks fast; has to speak very slowly. 19.

360. °Articulation and deglutition intensely painful. ⁰Diphtheria. 20.

°Breath very offensive. Diphtheria. 12, 17, 19, 21, 23, 26, 29, 32.

°Talking is very difficult, and there is a disposition to talk through nose. ⁰Nervous throat affection. 15.

No taste in mouth. 1 (4).

*Mouth constantly full of frothy saliva, but lips dry and parched. 1a (6).

Tongue coated white. 1a (5, 12, 13, 37).

Slight coating of tongue. 1a (7).

Tongue slightly coated white. 1a (8).

Tongue red and coated white. 1a (14).

Taste in the mouth as if she had been eating spoiled meat, increased by anything sweet, lasting all the morning. 1a (2).

370. Mucous in mouth, increased after *eating, and also in open air. 1a (5).

°Nothing tastes natural, except salt food. ⁰Epulis. 65.

°Mouth dry and parched. ⁰Diphtheria. 12.

°Tongue coated white in centre, edges red. ⁰Diphtheria. 12.

°Breath offensive, putrid. ⁰Diphtheria. 14.

°Breath tainted with diphtheritic odor. ⁰Diphtheria. 32.

THROAT.

Throat inflamed and painful. Sore greenish-yellow patch on r. side of throat, just above tonsil; pronounced "diphtheritic" by two allopathic physicians, who advised immediate cauterization. 1a (12).

*Roof of mouth and back wall of pharynx coated with a greyish-yellow deposit, the greater part of which soon disappeared, lasting only about an hour; (*Phyt.*) throat very much better by noon, deposit had nearly disappeared, but worse again by night. 1a (13).

*In morning throat very sore; r. tonsil covered with ulcers and patches, which extended over palate and covered l. tonsil (*Lyc.*); next day membrane extended across posterior wall of pharynx; uvula elongated, accompanied by chilliness, high fever, pains in head, back and limbs, great restlessness, and extreme prostration. An allopathic physician pronounced it severe "diphtheria," but it soon got well. 6.

380. Dark red angry streaks of capillaries flashing upward along faces of anterior pillars of fauces; the whole pharynx and fauces grew dark red and tumid; r. pillar covered with a dark-red eruption; l. tonsil has a small amount of swelling, and just above it, on the soft palate near the outer third of the arch, is a small round yellowish white spot, about a line in diameter, looking like the beginning of a diphtheritic patch; next day, spot on l. pillar of fauces larger, showing clearly that it is a true desquamation of epithelium, and identical with the pathological process in diphtheria; she feels precisely as she did when she had diphtheria last winter; in two days more the patch had disappeared, leaving reddened surface denuded of epithelium, and throat sore. 40 (5).

Burning in throat; Pharyngeal inflammation and rapid development on posterior surface of l. tonsil of a large thick yellowish patch, precisely similar in every particular to the appearance presented in her attack of malignant diphtheria last winter, (i. e., acute pharyngitis, face flushed, full bounding pulse, burning, smarting pain in throat, with ropy, slimy greenish-yellow offensive discharge, and later a pearly white membrane covering entire pharyngeal cavity.

°Small, round or irregular, grey white ulcers on tonsils and fauces, both sides. (*Merc. iod.*) °Diphtheria. 20.

°The diphtheritic patch appeared first on the r. tonsil, then on l., and frequently on alternated sides; the swelling of submaxillary and lymphatic cervical glands also alternated in like manner; there was a noticeable aggravation during and after a cold storm from the north-east. 14.

°Sore throat, ulcers on both tonsils, pain in front of trachæ on pressure. 14.

°White ulcers on tonsils. 12.

°As the cure progressed, and the membrane came off, throat became very painful, and he thought he was worse. 20.

°Dark and bleeding surface of throat, with patches and ulcers on both tonsils and fauces. 20.

°Right tonsil raw, swollen; grey-white membrane there and on fauces. °Diphtheria. 20, 26.

°The ulcers increase in size and number, but the neighboring membrane looks clearer. °Diphtheria. 20.

390. °Sore throat commencing on l. tonsil, which was swollen and ulcerated, and presented a depression covered by a white patch (*Lach.*); the disease later extended to palate and r. tonsil, the parts red and shining. 24, 26.

°Sore throat, ulcer on inner side of each tonsil, tonsils red and slightly enlarged, rest of throat dry. °Diphtheria. 19.

°Thick dirty-grey diphtheritic membrane covering free border of epiglottis, and extending off to each side. *Kali. bich*). 22.

°Uvula pretty free from membrane, but intensely sore and bleeds. °Diphtheria. 23.

°In most cases of diphtheria, the throat symptoms begin on r. side. 12.

°Throat covered with diphtheritic membrane; uvula elongated, swollen, and covered with black and white or grey diphtheritic deposit; back of throat, extending to hard palate, all covered; breath very offensive; l. side of neck swollen, and almost even with jaw (*Kali bich.*); great difficulty in swallowing; after throat began to improve, disease seemed to work through whole alimentary canal, for the vulva and parts were very much swollen, and every little while there would be involuntary discharges of diphtheritic matter from vulva and rectum. (*Apis.*) 19, 29.

°Many of the worst cases of diphtheria. 33, 34.

°Many cases of diphtheria and diphtheritic croup; also membranous croup. 18.

°Thick membranous mass lying on soft palate, l. side; diphtheritic masses covering uvula and posterior wall of throat; next day, membrane on soft palate thicker, dirty brown on uvula and posterior walls and pillars of throat, much more extensive and offensive; very difficult deglutition; a large membranous mass, which threatened suffocation, having been removed by forceps; on the following morning a second membrane had taken the place of the first, and the walls of throat were covered with a dirty-grey exudation; uvula almost black, and coarse shreds of membrane hanging from it. *Kali bich.*) 23.

°Tonsils swollen and diptheritic. 24.

400. Disease extending to palate and r. tonsil, which were red and shining. (*Canth. Puls.*) 24.

°Right tonsil covered with ash-grey membrane extending along free palatine border to uvula, which it had already involved; room loaded with diphtheritic odor; next day membrane had passed the centre, involving the whole arch of palate, and reaching far down on l. tonsil. 17.

°Whole of r. tonsil covered with diphtheritic patch. 21.

°On each tonsil a very thick exudation, covering nearly entire surface; while examining, a large piece of membrane was accidentally detached from one tonsil, followed by considerable hemorrhage. 16.

°Tongue, fauces, tonsils, all swollen, and covered with a dirty coating. θDiphtheria. 22.

°R. tonsil swollen, and on it a small diptheritic patch, the rest of throat being inflamed ; next morning both tonsils swollen and covered with diphtheritic patches, with difficult deglutition, which on sixth day had become impossible, refusing to drink, though complaining of intense thirst ; room filled with characteristic fetor ; membrane, swelling and soreness, most marked on r. side ; soreness of r. side now decreased, and commenced on l., the tonsil and posterior wall of pharynx being covered with the membrane, and the voice showing that it had involved the posterior nares. 21, 26.

°False membrane, thick-grey, yellow or dark, surrounding mucous membrane dark or bright, may be worse on either side, or inflammation shift from side to side, generally worse on l. 9.

°False membrane, thick, yellowish-grey, often greenish. 9.

°After membrane exfoliates, mucous membrane appears raw and bloody, with increased deglutition. 1.

°Whole membrane of throat swollen, dark red, with grey patches and small irregular-shaped ulcers ; membrane peeled off occasionally; articulation and deglutition intensely painful painful; worse after sleep. (*Lach.*) 20.

410. °False membrane in throat, thick grey, or slightly yellow, or dark and almost black, or white and glistening, almost like mother of pearl. 26.

°Sore throat, rapidly growing worse ; difficult swallowing, worse on r. side ; r. tonsil intensely inflamed, bright red and greatly enlarged, and a yellow-grey spot, the size of a dime, on inner surface; whole whole pharynx, uvula, and velum much inflamed ; next day, spot larger, and others forming in pharynx, and l. tonsil nearly as large as r.; almost total inability to swallow, especially liquids ; even a teaspoonful of water gave her much suffering ; characteristic fetor of breath. 31.

°Croupal diphtheria, with glossy shiny appearance of the bacteria, and a disposition of the membrane to change its position on fauces. 23.

°The white bacteria are smooth, shiny, glossy, and

readily disappear on one place to reappear just as rapidly on another part of throat. 13.

°In diphtheria, one side is attacked, and the pain leaves that side and is felt on the other, and so back and forth, the pain only on one side at a time. 14.

°In diphtheria, the ulcers go from one side to the other, and back again; the ulceration has a shining, glistening appearance (*Apis*); the swelling of the glands changes sides, and they are painful to touch. 14.

°Considerable difficulty in swallowing; uvula elongated and very much swollen, with diphtheritic coating on it; tonsils swollen and coated; back of throat patched, extending up to hard palate; odor offensive and diphtheritic. 19.

°Both tonsils swollen, and covered with spots of exudation, like the mould on preserves. 36.

°Throat sore, swollen, red, and glistening. θDiphtheria. 9.

°Throat highly inflamed, swollen, almost closed; grey diphtheritic spots on l. side of throat. 25.

420. °Sore throat, diphtheritic patches on l. side of throat and roof of mouth; could not swallow, had taken no food that night. 25.

°Whole membrane of throat highly inflamed, swollen, and glands enlarged on both sides. θDiphtheria. 25.

Tonsils inflamed and very sore. 2 (10).

°Tonsils swollen as almost to close the throat. θDiphtheria. 24.

°One or both tonsils swollen. θDiphtheria. 9.

°Enlarged tonsils, l. being the size of a small marble. θAfter diphtheria. 25.

°Sensation of rawness, commencing usually on l. side of throat. θDiphtheria. 9.

°Throat very much inflamed; tonsils swollen, l. nearly covered with diphtheritic patch or ulcer. 46.

°Quinsy; the suppuration ran from l. tonsil to r., then from r. to l., then back again to r., then both tonsils equally; and again one tonsil would improve and the other grow worse; the whole posterior portion of throat was an œdematous swelling, rising up like an insurmountable barrier; thick tough pieces of diphtheritic membrane were coming away, and new membranes constantly re-forming; the swelling in throat was so large and tense that the mouth could not be closed. 37.

°The diphtheritic deposits look as if varnished; exudations migratory, now here, now there. θDiphtheritic croup. 13.

430. °Dark red angry streaks of capillaries in fauces, giving place to a shining glistening deposit, or tough membrane; half-arches filled with sticky fetid saliva. 48.

°Throat sore, but little swelling, tonsils very slightly enlarged; soreness of throat first chiefly r., then l.; well marked diphtheritic membrane on both sides of throat situated on an inflamed red base, ¾ inch long, ¼ inch wide, ½ inch thick, and the same length and width as the base; anterior edge a dirty yellow; centre more organized, pearly, glistening, white like cartilage; membrane on right side seems more firm and dense, and disappeared later. 51.

°Throat very sore, tonsils enlarged, especially l., very large white patches; tonsils and pharynx deep purple red; putrid odor from throat; after the patches were expectorated, they left throat very sore, raw, and bloody. 12.

°Right tonsil red and swollen; pain in tonsil gnawing, worse at night; preventing sleep. 8.

10 p. m., throat feels dry and sore. (*Merc.*) 3a (1).

Slight nausea, and lips, mouth and throat dry and burning; next day the same, and woke in night with a very dry throat, and mouth and lips parched and burning. (*Arum tri.*) 3a (19).

Parched feeling in upper and back part of throat. (*Nux mos.*) 4 (1).

°Throat feels swollen and raw. (*Nux*). θDiphtheria. 24, 26).

Throat sore, with severe headache. (4).

Throat sore. 2 (5).

440. Throat sore, dry and hot. (*Bell.*) 2 (8).

Throat slightly sore. 1a (14, to 16, 18, 19 to 22, 34, 37).

Throat has a slight feeling of thickness in it; cannot call it a sore throat, and it causes no inconvenience. 39 (3).

⁰Pains in limbs, small of back, and head disappear; throat becomes more painful, but looks better. ᶿDiphtheria. 20 (of prover 64).

Soreness of throat directly under each ear, internally. 2 (3).

Throat slightly sore all the time; no particular spot, but all over. 1a (209 to 216.)

*Throat very sore, pain extending to chest; dry and sore; deep red color on either side of throat opposite tonsils: these symptoms continued, gradually decreasing till end of proving on 35th day. (*Merc.*) 2 (11, 12).

Throat slightly sore at sides. 2 (2).

Throat sore in afternoon and evening on r. side. 1a (7).

Throat very sore on r. side. 1a (13).

450. *Throat sore on l. side. (*Lach.*) 1e (5).

Throat well in morning, but a little sore on r. side in afternoon. 1a (17.)

Throat slightly sore on l. side for three days; the following day nearly well, quite well next day. 1a (23).

*Throat very sore on l. side; painful to external pressure both sides. 1e (12).

Throat sore, principally l. side; in three more days, still sore, but principally r. side; in three more days quite well. 1f (329).

⁰Sore throat on r. side, low down, and extending up to ear; pain when swallowing; sensitive to external pressure; slight coryza. (*Lach.*) 26 (1).

⁰Pain in throat pushes toward l. ear. ᶿDiphtheria. 20, 26.

⁰Sore spot in l. side of throat, only at night, removed by 1 m.; next night the same on r. side of throat; after 1 m. returned no more. 12, 26.

Throat feels raw and sore on r. side, with tickling sensation in throat. 1a (8).

⁰Tickling pain in throat when drinking. ᶿDiphtheria. 14.

460. ⁰Throat feels stiff. (*Lach.*) ᶿDiphtheria. 20, 26.

Raw sensation in back of throat. (*Lach.*) 1a (9).

Throat sore on l. side, with cough caused by irritation in upper part of throat, worse by lying down at night, after eating or drinking, and during and after talking; constant desire to urinate at the same time; soreness commenced with a tickling in throat, which caused constant coughing; came and went with menses. 1f (58).

**Throat commenced to be sore on l. side, and by night was so bad that she could scarcely swallow, which caused great pain; slight increase of saliva; next day throat nearly well in morning; by night quite well on l. side, but very sore on r.; which was covered with a greyish-yellow patch; subsequent day, throat well on r. side, but sore on l.; about twelve hours well on l. side but sore on r.; continued about twelve hours, then ceased, leaving her entirely free; all these throat symptoms ended, as they had begun, with menses. 1f (31).

***Soreness of throat commences with a tickling sensation, which causes constant cough; then a sensation of a lump on one side, causing constant deglutition: this condition entirely ceases, only to commence on the opposite side, and often alternates, again returning to its first condition; these sore throats are very apt to begin and end with menses. 1f (1873).

⁰Sore throat just before menses for several years ever since diphtheria; r. side of throat now worse, but it sometimes comes on one side, sometimes on the other; small yellowish white patches of exudation on tonsil of affected side, with great difficulty of swallowing, and sharp pains moving up into ear; these patches are also present on back of throat and uvula; some are quite yellow and some are white; scraping them off makes them bleed. 26.

⁰Throat has a burnt and drawn feeling as from caustic. ⁰Diphtheria. 24.

Throat feels *dry, husky, as if scalded by hot fluid. 40 (3).

Peculiar dryness of fauces and throat; sensation as if parched and swollen. (*Lach. Phos.*) 5.

In morning, smarting and burning in throat; through the day made many and loud complaints about throat. 41 (2).

470. ⁰Pricking sensation in throat, as if full of sticks. (*Hep.*) 12, 26.

^{0}Pricking and cutting pains shoot through l. tonsil when swallowing. (*Nit.ac.*) $^{\theta}$Diphtheria. 24.

^{0}Pricking and cutting pains through tonsils when swallowing. $^{\theta}$Diphtheria. 26, 29.

^{0}Pricking, cutting pains on swallowing. 9.

^{0}Pricking and cutting pains on swallowing, shooting up to ears. $^{\theta}$Diphtheria. 26.

Occasional slight probing pains in l. lower throat. 44 (11).

Feeling of a *lump in throat, which goes down when swallowing, but returns; throat worse r. side; worse on swallowing saliva: afterwards, throat which had been getting well, suddenly one evening grew rapidly worse, but this time on l. side. 43 (19).

^{0}Sensation of a ball or round body in l. side of throat, and a feeling that it could be removed with a knife. 27.

^{0}Marked sensation of lump in throat on l. side, when swallowing, and the pain from the act extended to l. ear. $^{\theta}$Diphtheria. 21, 26.

^{0}Most pain when swallowing solids, no aversion to cold drink; when swallowing solid food, it seems to pass over a lump, with sore and aching pains extending to and in l. ear. $^{\theta}$Diphtheria. 24.

^{0}Sensation as though there was a lump in r. upper part of throat. 1a (17) 1d (2).

^{0}Lump on l. side of pharynx below tonsil, causing an enlargement that filled each arch of palate, nearly to r. side. 12.

^{0}Gargling with warm water brought up a little stringy mucous. $^{\theta}$Diphtheria. 24.

Great dryness of throat, with secretion of thick viscid saliva in throat, so tough and tenacious that it must be wiped away with a handkerchief, since it cannot be expectorated. 40 (5).

Great dryness of tonsils in night, preceded during day by large collections of mucous in throat. Dryness and hurting of the throat, peculiar, felt like she did when she had diphtheria last winter. 40 (4).

Slight throat irritation on l. side; urging to hawk, principally morning. 44 (3).

°Throat worse by empty swallowing. (*Ignat.*) θDiphtheria. 20.

°Throat relieved after drinking cold or warm. θDiphtheria. 20.

Not much pain on swallowing after third day of illness. θDiphtheria. 9.

°Refuses all fruit, berries, oranges, because they make throat smart. °Diphtheria. 19.

490. °Would desist and cry at every attempt to nurse, and reach for water, yet refuse to take it. θDiphtheria. 22.

*Pain in upper and r. side of pharynx. 1c (17).

*Pain in r. side of throat in region of tonsil; nothing abnormal visible. θAcute rheumatism. 14.

Tonsils sore and irritated. 2 (9).

Tonsils and throat quite sore. 2 (10).

*Left tonsil feels sore. 2 (1).

°Sensation of a lump in r. side of throat, with a feeling that she could take hold of it with her fingers and pull it out; accompanied by a very annoying pricking, stitching feeling; constant inclination to swallow saliva, which caused soreness of throat. 27.

Passage of particles of food into opening of posterior nares, lodging and remaining for hours apparently just above the free border of soft palate; uvula elongated and smartly curved with the convexity toward l. side; muscular tissue of l. half of velum pendulum palate was paretic; at meals his mind was fixed upon hs tihroat, and he watched for the crumbs of food that, despite all his care, would go up instead of down. 30.

°Sensation as if throat were closing and she would choke, the sensation is between throat and nose; feels as if something in throat were either enlarged or relaxed; desires to keep mouth open lest she should choke; sometimes cannot swallow, because there seems to be a kind of muscular contraction in throat. 15.

°Almost total inability to swallow, especially liquids; even a teaspoonful of water gave her much suffering. θDiphtheria. 31.

500. °Swallowing almost impossible. °Diphtheria. 24.

°Great difficulty in swallowing. °Diphtheria. 12, 19, 21, 23, 24, 25, 26, 29, 31.

°Very difficult deglutition, but little pain. °Diphtheria. 23.

°Child refuses to swallow water, and sputters out the medicine, some returning by the nose. Diphtheria. 22.

°Could swallow only with great difficulty, though anæsthesia of throat continued as before. Diphtheria. 23.

°Swallowing very painful. Diphtheria. 20, 23, 12.

*Constant inclination to swallow. 1a (5, 7, 13. 18).

*Constant inclination to swallow, which causes pain extending to r. ear. 1c (17).

°Constant inclination to swallow, which causes pain extending to both ears. 26.

°Constant inclination to swallow, though deglutition is painful. °Diphtheria. 9.

510. Throat sore to external pressure on. r side. 1e (15).

°Throat very sensitive to touch externally. (*Lach.*) °Diphtheria. 9, 16, 22, 26.

°External swelling l. side, not much soreness on swallowing, but whole side very sensitive to touch. °Diphtheria. 23.

°Swelling of l. parotid, with sore throat and loss of appetite. 29.

Swelling of r. submaxillary gland with considerable soreness, almost well next day ; on subsequent day swelling of l. submaxillary gland with much soreness, which was still sore and swollen on following day. 1a (29).

°Glandular (parotid) swelling passes from l. to r. 20.

°Swelling of cervical and submaxillary glands. °Diphtheria. 9.

°Throat worse at one time on r. side, at another on l. °Diphtheria. 26.

°Submaxillary glands swollen. °Diphtheria. 24.

°Inflamation and swelling shift from side to side, generally worse on l. Diphtheria. 9, 26.

520. °Throat sore, œdematous, puffed, tonsils badly swollen. 16.

°If the parotid glands are first attacked, and the disease extends to other glands of neck; throat and sides of neck not tender to external touch. Diphtheria. 13.

°Throat sensitive. Parenchymatous metritis. 32.

°Deglutition exceedingly difficult and painful. Diphtheria. 12.

°Some redness of l. side of throat, but no sensation of soreness, increased next day ; on subsequent day, redness of throat increased, with a slight sensation of soreness on r. side. 1a (2).

*Throat slightly sore on r. side. 1a (5).

*Throat feels raw. 1a (5).

*Tickling sensation in throat. 1a (8).

Tickling and *sense of contriction in upper part of throat, causing *constant dry hacking cough. 1a (9).

°Wakes with throat and mouth painfully dry. °Parenchymatous metritis. 32.

530. In morning, began to feel a sore place, like a sore boil, on l. tonsil ; not quite so sore in evening, though the back was more painful ; not felt much next night. 62 (4).

On waking in morning throat felt as if there were lumps in it like two eggs, and sore *all the time, especially *when swallowing anything ; *cold water seemed to relieve momentarily ; in evening, examination revealed both tonsils *much swollen and very red, l. *most ; and distinct *patches on l. tonsil. 62 (5).

Shortly before retiring to bed, throat began to feel *raw and sore; did not sleep well that night; next morning, throat felt *full and sore, and a little the worse on r. side; this condition continued two days, when it seemed to *continue downwards to chest. 63 (7).

°On swallowing, acute pain at one time on r. side of throat, and again on l. side. °Diphtheria. 14.

°Throat very dry and sore, much inflamed, worse on r. side ; palate red, uvula elongated; very painful deglutition. 12.

°Sore throat, pains in whole body and limbs, severe headache. °Diphtheria. 12.

°Throat very sore, worse on l. side ; large greenish

ulcers on both tonsils, surrounded by grey-white exudation, the parts not covered are a deep purple red; swelling externally on both sides; after exudation on tonsils disappeared, a raw bloody surface was left. [θ]Diphtheria. 12.

[0]Membrane would leave throat, and a very severe interstitial hemorrhage of bright red blood would ensue; the hemorrhage would slowly improve, and the membrane appear again in throat; these had continued to alternate for several days. [θ]Diphtheria. 68.

[0]Throat became bad, deglutition difficult; mucous follicles raised or swollen, and covered with a whitish cream-colored mucous. 32.

For about two weeks had sore throat all the time, diagnosed by Dr. B. as diphtheritic. 1f (Oct., 1873.)

540. [0]White patches, like eggs of flies) on both tonsils, extending thence to back of throat; tonsils enlarged and deep red; felt she would suffocate at night from full feeling in throat which prevented sleep; swallowing toast gave some pain, but seemed to clear the throat; drinking anything caused more pain in throat, and she had to gulp it down. 15.

[0]A serious case of quinsy, just ready to discharge, disappeared without discharging, in an unusually short time; the guiding symptoms were the trouble changing from one side to the other and back again; the relief was within a few minutes, and the quinsy has not returned. 73.

Throat relieved by eating. 1a (12).

Throat inflamed and painful. 1a (12).

[0]Ulcers on throat shine like silver gloss, symptoms went from side to side; croupy symptoms not well marked; after exudation was cleared off, a deep excavation was left. [θ]Diphtheria. 75. Authority, J. A. Wakeman, M. D.

[0]Throat filled with substance that looked like what Germans call "smear kase." Throat, tongue, roof of mouth, gums and cheeks completely lined with this substance. Mouth and throat filled with loose particles; it had a horrible odor. [θ]Post-scarletina diphtheria. 76 (sixth trituration.) Authority, W. B. Stover, M. D.

STOMACH.

Appetite improved. 2 (4).

Appetite increased. 1a (12).

Vigorous appetite. 2 (9).

Cannot satisfy her hunger. 1a (14).

Very hungry all day, cannot eat enough to satisfy herself; feels as hungry after eating as before. (*Cascar. Calc. Chinin. Cina. Lyc. Strout.*) 1a (13).

Thought dinner-time (noon) would never come; voracious hunger and he sat down to eat; the hunger left him and he could eat nothing. 38 (2).

Appetite good; eats until ashamed of herself, and leaves the table with a desire to eat as much more, though she has no hunger till she sees the food. 1c (379).

550. The appetite, usually poor, has been greatly increased during the proving. 1.

Almost all desire for food has been gone, but now can scarcely get enough to satisfy her ; could eat at least six times a day. 1e (319).

*Desire for highly-seasoned dishes, which is very unusual ; has used pepper, mustard and salt freely. 1e (379).

Has had a great repugnance to meat, could not eat a mouthful of it; but now has a great craving for it. 1e (319).

Great disinclination to eat anything; yet as soon as she commences, the dislike passes off and the food tastes good. 1e (209 to 216).

*No appetite. 2 (11). Diphtheria. 21, 16, 19, 46. $^{\theta}$Acute rheumatism. 52.

No appetite for meat. 3 (6).

No appetite for supper; in two days appetite still growing less, little appetite for breakfast, but feels chiefly in forenoon ; in four days completely lost; in seven days re-gaining it ; in ten days poor. 44 (3).

^{0}No appetite, cannot bear food. $^{\theta}$Dyspepsia. 25.

^{0}Great difficulty in getting her to take nourishment. $^{\theta}$Diphtheria. 19.

560. ^{0}Great indisposition to take food or drink. $^{\theta}$Tonsillitis. 16.

*Considerable thirst. 1a (9).

Very thirsty. 1a (20).

Thirst. 1a (22, 30).

°Great thirst for large quantities, often. (*Nat. Mur.*) 12, 26.

Great thirst for very cold water in small quantities, which causes teeth to ache. 1a (19).

Wants to drink very cold water all the time, only in very small quantities. 1a (8).

°Thirst frequent for small quantities. (*Arsen. Act.*). 12. °Diphtheria. 12.

°Thirst changeable. °Diphtheria. 9.

°Aversion to liquids, especially water. °Diphtheria. 31.

°Desire for warmish water with a pinch of salt in. Diphtheria. 9.

°Thirst. °Acute rheumatism. 52.

570. °Appetite and strength failing; dislike to food, especially fat or greasy. °Parenchymatous metritis. 32.

°Entire loss of appetite; obliged to take liquid food. °Parenchymatous metritis. 32

°Craves milk and drinks much of it. °Diphtheria. 12.

Eructations of tasteless gas. 1a (6).

Dizzy, nausea, as after rich food, worse after standing, must sit down, feels as if she would fall if she closed her eyes ; seven days the same nausea. 43 (1).

Nausea while in bed, worse by motion, lasting all the morning. 1a (6).

Nausea, with *headache, on waking; continuing all the morning. 1 (11).

Nausea from leaning forwards. 1a (25).

Nausea on first rising. (*Lyc. Magn. m. Mang. Puls. Rhus. Sab. Trios.*) 1a (14).

Considerable nausea. 1a (12).

580. Slight nausea, aggravated by moving around, relieved by keeping quiet; during menses. 3a (17).

Nausea relieved by eructations of wind. 1d (1).

Stomach out of order: slight nausea on rising at 7 p. m. 2 (3).

At 10 a. m. slight nausea, lasting only a few minutes. 3 (15).

Slight nausea while dressing in morning. 3a (8).

At 10 p. m. slight nausea with thirst. 4 (3).

At 5 p. m. while smoking a cigar, great nausea with severe pain in stomach-pit; vomiting seemed imminent, but the sensation ceased in 4 or 5 minutes, and did not return. (*Tabac*). 4 (9).

Gagging from sore tonsils. 2 (9).

Sick at stomach, vomiting hard ; went home to bed. 2 (21).

⁰The almost constant diphtheretic discharges from mouth and nose nearly ceased, and she almost immediately had spells of sickness of stomach, and would occasionally vomit pieces of membrane. θDiphtheria. 19.

590. ⁰Nausea at beginning of diphtheria. (3 cases). 36.

⁰Great faintness of stomach and nausea. θParenchymatous metritis. 32.

At 10-15 a. m., *empty, weak feeling in stomach pit ; next day the same at 6 p. m. (*Dig. Ign. Petrol. Sep.*). 3 (3).

Before dinner, a very week feeling in stomach-pit. 3a (7).

Weak *sinking feeling in stomach-pit, on waking in morning. 1a (8).

A growling and disturbed state of stomach. 2 (8).

Pain with flatulence, in epigastric region. 7 (2).

At 9-45 p. m., dyspeptic pain, *as from a stone, or undigested food, in stomach pit; followed by a stabbing pain in r. lung, just below nipple. (*Kali. bich.*) 4 (1).

⁰Stomach tender and bloated; cannot eat or drink anything without pain in stomach-pit. θAfter Diphtheria. 25.

⁰Burning in epigastric region, feeling of a weight and pressure of a stone in stomach. 25.

600. ⁰Severe throbbing in region of solar plexus; when it becomes very severe, which it did daily for hours at a time, it would seem to extend or continue upwards to head, when dizziness and lightness of head would supervene, requiring her to lie down at once, otherwise she would fall violently to the floor. 27.

⁰Gastralgia or cardialgia, worse at menses, so she would drop to the floor, comes and goes suddenly. 47.

°Beating in stomach and bowels. °Parenchymatous metritis. 32.

°No appetite or thirst. °Diphtheria. 46.

Very hungry; could not eat enough to satisfy herself. 1a (19).

Aversion to anything sweet. 1a (3, 8).

In stomach, feeling as if something were pushing up. 43 (8).

°Frequent attacks of severe vomiting, and when not so, always feeling of nausea, and fear to eat. °Sick headache. 15.

°Thirst for little at a time, but often, as throat is so dry and hot. °Diphtheria. 12.

Sinking, gone sensation in stomach-pit. 20.

°Gnawing, hungry feeling, not relieved by eating; every thing she eats, except fish, makes her worse: the thought of milk makes her sick, since sick headache was cured can now eat anything. °Sick headache. 77. Authority J. T. Kent, M. D.

ABDOMEN AND HYPOCHONDRIA.

610. Pain in r. side of pelvis; while it lasted there was no pain in l. side. 1a (22).

Sharp contractive pain just in front of r. anterior superior spine of ilium, lasting all day, sometimes occurring very frequently and then leaving possibly for half an hour; pain of the same character but not exactly like it, in l. ovarian region. 1e (382).

°Severe burning pain in r. hypochondriac and iliac region and corresponding part of back, extending across back to l. side of abdomen; worse when on the feet or when fatigued, better when lying down. 10.

Low down in r. groin, above ramus, three lancinations up toward crest of ilium, waking her from sleep. 71 (3).

°Smarting in r. groin; pains seem to be in pelvic bones, uterus, and limbs. °Parenchymatous metritis. 32

Burning in l. side of pelvis. (*Amm. c. Graph. Plat. Ruta. Sep.*) 1a (20).

Sensation of extreme heat in l. side of abdomen and pelvis. not confined to any one spot. but general. 1a (37).

Pain and burning in l. side of abdomen and pelvis, with weight and dragging on that side : the clothes feel very heavy 1a (21).

Pressure and pain in l. side of pelvis. 1a (25).

Intense sharp pains in l. side of abdomen with nausea, caused by leaning forwards. 1a (17).

620. Pain in l. side of abdomen and pelvis all the morning. 1a (38).

Pulsative boring pain in abdomen, to l. of umbilicus, for several days. 1f (Aug. 1873).

Rumbling and gurgling in l. lower abdomen. 1a (b).

Feeling of tension in l. groin; does not want to walk or stand, as it increases the sensation ; relieved by flexing leg on abdomen. 1a (18).

During afternoon, uneasy pain in l. groin; returning the following afternoon. and lasting till 10 p. m. 44 (18).

Sharp pain in l. side of abdomen, in front of ilium : the pressure of clothes was painful: entirely removed by loosening them. 1.

Sharp pain in l. anterior superior spinous process of ilium, during expiration. 1a (38).

Pains and tension in l. groin. 1a (19).

°Very acute pain in l. groin, extending up l. side to crest of ilium: relieved by stool; sometimes the pain is in track of colon. 1.

Pain passing from crest of l. ilium to l. ovarian region. 1a (62).

630. *During evening, slight sensation of pressure in abdomen and pelvis, from within outwards. 1 (62).

*Slight pain in l. side of abdomen and pelvis, lasting only a few minutes. 1a (62).

Abdomen swollen and hard. (*Calc. c. Sach. Alb. Sep.*). 1a (16).

Abdomen swollen and very hard. 1a (37).

*In evening, abdomen very hard and swollen. 1a (44).

Abdomen hard, and sensitive to deep pressure. 1a (15).

Abdomen swollen, and sensitive to deep pressure, which

also causes nausea, the nausea passes off when pressure is relieved. 1a (17).

[0]Abdomen swollen and burning, with bearing-down pains therein. 25.

Feeling of uneasiness in umbilical region, an agitation or moving as it were, in the colon about this part. 44 (3).

Pain in lower abdomen like a stoppage there, always about 2 a. m. relieved by passage of flatus downwards. 54 (6, 7).

640. Rumbling and gurgling in abdomen, with escape of flatus. 1a (33).

Rumbling in bowels with passing of flatus in morning, soon followed by a copious liquid stool, accompanied by a peculiar nervous tremor all over body, with slight tingling to ends of fingers: there was no second discharge. 7 (6).

Woke at 2.30 a. m., with intense pain in abdomen, and desire for stool which could hardly be supressed; after repairing to closet, the diarrhoeic stool was voided entire at one effort, and ease immediately secured. 44 (5).

Felt as though abdomen and chest were firmly compressed all over, as if the skin were contracted. 1c (21).

Sharp shooting pains in abdomen and pelvis, worse on l. side. 1a (13).

Severe shooting pains in abdomen and pelvis, passing in all directions. 1a (33).

In evening, pain in upper abdomen as of wind. 4 (2).

Colicky pains and wind in bowels, with restlessness during night. (*Nat. Nit.*) 4 (3).

Slight pain in upper abdomen. 4 (4).

Abdomen very sensitive to pressure. (*Puls. Sulp.*) 1a (13).

650. Abdomen very sensitive to pressure and weight of clothes, entirely relieved by removing them, during very profuse menses. 1d (6).

Pressure of clothes causes intense pain and distress in abdomen. (*Act. Rau. bulb.*) 1d (7).

Abdomen painful from the least weight of hand or arm.

1a (38).

*Pains in abdomen intermittent. 1a (16)

Fine miliary eruption on abdomen, preceded by nausea and pains in abdomen. 72.

*Pain in pelvis, principally in r. ovarian region. (*Apis. Pallad.*) 1a (17).

*Headache over l. eye on first waking, and great pain in pelvis, most marked at r. ovary. 1a (18).

Slight pain across bowels. 2 (2).

Slight pain across bowels in morning. 2 (6).

Pains in abdomen caused by leaning forward. 1a (12, 14).

660. Pains in abdomen relieved by leaning back. 1a (16, 37).

Abdomen and pelvis extremely hot. 1a (15).

Burning sensation in pelvis, with pains in all directions. (*Camph. Nitr. Phos. ac. Stram.*) 1a (14).

Burning sensation in lower part of abdomen and pelvis, passing from side to side. 1a (13).

During afternoon, burning sensation all across pelvis, particularly on l. side, with considerable pain. 1a (18).

Constant pains across lower part of abdomen. 1d (22).

Slight pressure in abdomen from within outwards. 1a (13).

Outward pressure in abdomen and pelvis. 1a (19).

Great pressure in abdomen from within outwards. 1a (20).

Pressure in abdomen from within outwards. 1a (37).

670. *Pressure from within outwards, as if the contents of of abdomen would be forced outwards literally, just above pelvis. 1a (14).

The contents of abdomen and pelvis seem as though they were coming out just above the pelvis. 1a (21).

Cutting pains in lower part of abdomen. 1a (37).

Abdomen very hard and feels as if it would burst. 1a (18).

Sensation while walking as if abdomen would burst. (*Lyc.*) 1a (17).

Abdomen feels as though it would burst. 1c (6).

Pain in l. side of pelvis. 1a (22).

Weight and dragging in l. side of pelvis. 1a (22).

Pain in l. side of pelvis, weight and dragging on that side. 1a (23).

Sharp pains in all directions on l. side of pelvis, worse by pressure. 1a (6).

680. Pain in lower part of abdomen and pelvis, on l. side; increased by pressure of arm or hand. 1a (44).

Tension of l. groin relieved by drawing the leg up to body. 1a (21).

Feeling of tension in l. groin. 1a (22).

Pains in abdomen and pelvis. 1a (36).

Pressure of arm or hand increases the abdominal pain. 1a (37).

Great distress all over abdomen and pelvis, slight relief by leaning back. 1c. (6).

Menstruation at various times was preceded by an accession of flatulence. 1.

During evening, slight sensation of pressure in abdomen and pelvis from within outwards. 1a (62).

Riding in a carriage seems to jar her, and seems to increase the abdominal pain, while walking does not influence it in any way. 1a (13).

Clothes feel very heavy. 1a (13).

690. Abdomen and pelvis extremely hot. 1a (15).

Slight pain very low down in abdomen, during menses. 3a (15). (see under HEAD).

Rumbling in abdomen, which is slightly distended. 1c (209 to 216).

RECTUM AND STOOL.

Frequent and ineffectual urging to stool, with much straining. (*Lach. Nux. Sulph*). But neither constipation or diarrhœa. 1a (5).

The frequent desire for stool has been very annoying all through the provings. 1.

Frequent and urgent desire for stool; sensation as if the stool could not be evacuated on account of its great size and hardness: great pressure all across perineum; it is possible this was *retroversion of uterus as no stool followed the attempt. (*Bry. Kali.*) 1c (319).

When having a soft passage there is great tenesmus: the rectum does not act as if it had lost power, but as if it could not expel foeces because they are soft, and adhere to the parts like clay. (*Plat.*) 1e (209 to 216).

Tenesmus, but the stool was of ordinary consistency. 1e (395).

⁰Obstinate constipation ; frequent desire with darting pains in rectum, no power to expel; stool large, whitish, rough, scaly, hard. ⁰Diphtheria. 14.

*Constipation. 2 (2). ⁰Acute rheumatism. 52.

700. First movement of bowels for four days. 4 (12).

Slightly constipated: occasionally natural passages ; urgent desire for stool, but passes nothing but wind, or possibly one or two small pieces like sheep-dung: considerable wind in abdomen, with rumbling but never any pain. 1c (209 to 216).

Slight diarrhœa. 2 (5).

Profuse diarrhœa, with colic pain: diarrhœa watery, profuse, coming out with great force. 12.

⁰Mucous yellow liquid stools. 25.

Diarrhœa coming on promptly every evening at 9 p.m. (11).

Bowels relaxed, with frequent desire for stool ; acute transient pain in bowels. 4 (7).

At 5.30 a. m., fruitless attempt at stool, terminating in profuse evacuation, with but very little pain at 6.30 a. m. 4 (3).

Since the proving, the bowels act night and morning ; previously at night only. 2.

Constant pricking sensation at anus, lasting all the morning. 1a (6).

710. Great constipation before and after menses ; bowels very loose (not diarrhœa) during menses. 1e (June, 1872).

Very watery diarrhœa, only in morning. 1a (33).

Diarrhœa, very watery discharge, with much pressure at anus. 1a (6).

URINE.

Pain in urethra during urination, and lasting for a short time afterwards. 1a (12).

Urination causes intense pain in urethra, soon passing

off. 1a (13).

Sensation after urinating, as though the bladder were still full. (*Calc. c., Con. Ruta*). 1a (30).

Very sharp pain in bladder ten minutes after urinating, aggravated by pressure. (*Berb., Canth., Nat.mur.*) 3 (18).

After urination, continued desire to urinate. (*Calc. Con. Guiac. Laur. Ruta.*) 3 (18).

Emission of a drop or two after urinating. (*Lach. Petr.*) 1 (30).

After urination, a few more drops dribble out; to her great discomfort. 1f (6).

720. Frequent desire to urinate, which if not immediately attended to, causes pain in region of bladder. (*Puls*). The pain is a numb, dull sensation; if it is not relieved by urination it spreads over abdomen and l. side to ends of fingers ; never in head ; would frequently wake at night dreaming of the pain, and would have to urinate to relieve it. 1e (May, 1872).

Very frequent desire to urinate, passing a large quantity in proportion to the water drunk. 1f (76).

Constant desire to *urinate, easily restrained ; frequent urination, quantity variable, light colored, rather scanty. 1c (3).

Constant inclination to urinate ; urine profuse, natural color. 1a (52).

°Constant desire to urinate, with intense pain. °Urethral chancre. 14.

*Constant desire to urinate. 1a (20, 21, 53, 61); 5 after 40 M, 18 after 40 m, 11 after CM). Parenchymatous metritis. 32.

Constant inclination to *urinate, the inclination does not abate by urinating. 1a (65).

Constant desire to *urinate, urine scanty and frequent. 1b (2).

*Constant desire to urinate, urine scanty. 1c (6).

*Constant inclination to urinate, which was restrained as urination caused intense pain when coming in contact with vulva. 1c (20).

730. Occasionally very frequent urination, sometimes scalding the parts as it flows over them, yet not producing any soreness. 1e (June, 1872).

Constant and urgent desire to urinate; urine scanty and very light-colored. 1c (10).

*Constant desire to urinate, passing large quantities frequently; at night she dreams of urinating, and wakes to find an immediate necessity (*Kreos.*); a less strong and healthy person would probably have wet the bed. 1e (209 to 216).

Very sharp constant distressing pain in bladder, with frequent uncontrollable urging and tenemus; emptying bladder does not help, though it seems as if it would; this pain lasted fifteen hours, gradually diminishing as it passed away. 40 (3).

*Urine frequent and profuse. (*Merc.*, *Nat.m.*) 1a (30); 3a (1).

Frequent urination, quantity variable, light-colored. 1.

Urine frequent; profuse, light-colored. 1a (23, 28).

*Urine frequent, scanty, high colored. 1a (8).

Urination frequent and scanty. 1a (18).

Urination frequent, scanty, *high colored, red sediment. 1a (22).

Constant urination. 6.

740. °Urine high-colored or dark, plentiful, but passed at long intervals. 9.

°Urine frequent, especially at night. 1a (24).

°Plentiful discharge of urine, clear or high-colored, at long intervals. °Diphtheria. 9.

Urination has been especially troublesome at *night, causing her to wake two or three times every night to urinate. 1.

Urine strong and high-colored. 2 (12).

°Urine very scanty and dark. °Acute rheumatism. 14.

°Urine partially suppressed. °Tonsilitis. 16.

°Urine dark, with frequent urination. °Diphtheria. 20.

°Urine scanty, infrequent, coffee-colored, no desire to urinate, quantity less than a gill in twenty-four hours, eighty per cent. albumen, with much mucous. °Diphtheria. 14.

Urine *dark, heavily loaded with thick reddish sediment that adhered in different colored circles to bottom and sides of vessel. 44 (7).

750. °Great difficulty in urinating. °Diphtheria. 19.

°Urinating only once in twenty-four hours, and then

very copiously, but with some difficulty and slight irritation. °Diphtheria. 19.

°No urine for forty-seven and three-quarter hours, bladder pretty full, parts fearfully swollen, and irritation on urination very great. °Diphtheria. 19.

Woke frequently in night to urinate, and complained of great vesical tenismus, with sharp steady pain that made her weep and complain almost all night. 41 (2).

Frequent and very profuse urination; no thirst. 1d (14).

°Urine bright colored. °Diphtheria. 12.

°Slight difficulty in urinating, but at times very profuse and light-colored. °Parenchymatous metritis. 32.

D esire to urinate often, with difficulty. °Parenchymatous metritis. 32.

*Urine unusually frequent and dark. 62 (5).

Constant and urgent inclination to urinate in large quantities, though not at all thirsty; urine high colored; next day, the same urgent inclination, but urine was scanty, very turbid, and left a reddish sediment. 1e (209 to 216).

760\. Nocturnal enuresis, a specific. 25.

Urine painful and passing in drops. 28.

MALE SEXUAL ORGANS.

Sexual desire quite marked. 44 (7).

R. spermatic cord, low down, sore to touch. 44 (16).

°Buboes and chancres. 12.

Chancre on prepuce, l. side of frenum, granulating rapidly from centre to circumference. 12.

At 8 p.m., considerable itching and burning for ten minutes; near glans where formerly a chancre had existed, after eight days more, the same at 10 p. m., lasting much longer; after eleven days the same in forenoon, the part red and feverish; after twelve days, itching and redness; and after fifteen days, at 9 p. m., itching, with boring, throbbing pain. 44 (2).

°Large chancre on dorsum penis, with a fungoid bacterie mass covering the whole of the corona glandis, which was first of a glossy, shining, white appearance, and later covered with a fungus, looking like fully developed aphthæ; the edges of the swollen prepuce were covered with nodosities and itching. 13.

⁰Penis enormously swollen, chancre on glands, no pain; chancre was like a cauliflower excrescence, over half inch in diameter, red, smooth, and glistening. Gave 30th potency. In a week two more small chancres, deep sharp edges, clean, with the same shining appearance. Cm. cured. 14.

⁰Small sore at entrance of urethra; kept getting worse; prepuce involved for about half inch, and the parts of glans around urethra an open ulcer, exhaling the most fetid smell, and with most excruciating pain; hemorrhage at 10 p. m. every evening, and during the day when removing the dressings; constant desire to urinate, with intense pain; no sleep for a fortnight, red glistening appearance. 14.

770. ⁰Gonorrhœal pains, intermittent, in front, middle, or posterior part of urethra. 14.

⁰When the gonorrhœa is better, catarrh sets in. 14.

Female Sexual Organs.

Menses scanty; terribly cross and impatient first day; on second day, severe paroxysmal pains in uterine region, causing nausea; occasional pain in l. ovarian region, passing about half way down thigh, on upper part of it; all these pains better by bending backwards; pain and aching in r. lumbar region when leaning forwards (as in sewing) even for a short time; entire relief when bending back. 1e (371, 372).

Menses commence at regular period, scanty at first, with considerable pain in region of l. ovary. (*Arg.*, *Lach.*, *Thuj.*) 1d (5).

Menses for last few months (though now normal) have had a very strong ammoniacal smell, and wash out very easily; at the close the smell was horrible, ammonia being the most prominent, and stains a dark olive-green. 1c (June, 1872).

Menses three days in advance. 3 (51).

At 7 a. m., menses commence three days in advance, very free flow, no pain, feels well. 3 (26).

Menses commence three days too soon; flow very scanty and intermittent.

Menses bright red ; when put into water, the blood forms into long strings, which soon dissolve; passage of several small pieces of thin white transparent substance, having a distinctly organized structure, but extremely delicate ; next day flow more profuse, and the blood natural in character ; menses last four days. 1a (15).

Menses seven days too soon ; flow came in gushes, scanty, intermittent, *bright red, and *stringy, preceded by much flatulence from bowels. 1a (37).

Menses four days too soon, scanty but otherwise normal; 1a (62)

780. Menses commenced seven days too soon, very scanty. 1c (5).

°Menses fourteen days too soon, profuse. 14.

Menses every two weeks, accompanied by lassitude, pains in uterine region, and slight headache. 1f (Aug. 1873).

Menses very profuse and gushing. 1d (7 to 11).

Menses very profuse ; abdomen very sensitive to pressure and weight of clothes, entire relief by removing them. 1d (6).

Menses more profuse, but not as much as is natural ; somewhat *stringy. 1a (38).

Menses commenced scanty, and accompanied by slight feeling of distress in abdomen, ' 1a (210).

°Menses too early and too profuse, with bright-red blood. changing soon to dark clots and stringy; preceded by great engorgment of the breasts, with great sensitiveness to touch. 26.

Menses commence, flow very slight in amount for three days; next day very profuse, almost like flooding. 1e (15).

°Most excellent in Dysmenorrhœa. 16. °Parenchymatous metritis. 32.

790. °Several cases of membranous dysmenorrhœa. 33.

Uterine hemorrhage, when blood is bright-red and stringy. 26.

Dysmenorrhœa, pain in l. groin, with bearing down and nervousness. (Two cases). 36.

Discharge of blood from vagina all day, scanty, and bright. 1d (22).

Pressure on vulva causes a slight flow of blood. 1d (27 - 9).

Every evening after dinner, from Sept. 5th to 11th, when menstruation commenced, there was a slight discharge of blood which could be increased by pressure on the vulva. 1e (39 to 45).

Leucorrhœa only while standing. 1a (34).

Leucorrhœa all the afternoon. 1a (12).

Leucorrhœa at night, none in day. 1a (28).

*Leucorrhœa all day, but none at night, even after taking a long walk. 1a (7).

800. Leucorrhœa during day. 1a (8).

Leucorrhœa at night. 1a (29).

*Leucorrhœa lasting all day, but ceasing after 6 p.m., worse when standing or walking. 1a (5).

Leucorrhœa. 1a (6).

*Slight leucorrhœa during day, worse when standing or walking. 1a (20).

Slight leucorrhœa. (1a 13, 14).

*Slight watery leucorrhœa. 3 (61); 3a (1).

Slight watery leucorrhœa which stains but little. 3 (8).

⁰Leucorrhea, very profuse during day, none at night; discharge whitish and watery; pain in small of back; very irritable. 36.

Leucorrhœa continuing many days in succession. 1.

810. Leucorrhœa, worse about menstrual period. 29.

Leucorrhœa appeared instead of menses. 55.

*Severe pain in r. ovarian region, completely relieved by a flow of bright-red blood which lasted for about an hour; and did not return. 1a (26). 11 (356).

*In the afternoon, sharp pains in r. ovarian region, not constant but intermittent. (*Apis.*) 1a (38).

Constant pain in r. ovarian region. 1c (5).

Constant pain all day in region of r. ovary. 1c (6).

Constant pain in l. ovarian region. 1c (7).

⁰Sharp pain in r. ovary. 36.

Constant pain in l. ovary. (*Arg. Lach.*) 1 (6 after 40 m).

*Pain in l. ovarian region. 1a (37).

820. *Pain in l. ovarian region, and all across lower part of abdomen. 1a (38).

⁰Sharp pains beginning in l. ovary, and darting like lightning either towards r. ovarian region, or else

up l. side and down arm, or sometimes down both thighs; but most generally down l. leg to foot, which is numb; pains act something like labor-pains, and are accompanied by great restlessness of legs and arms, and great aching in lumbar region; on fifth day after premature labor. 26.

⁰Severe pain in entire uterine region, with profuse discharge of yellow, brown, and bloody leucorrhœa, two weeks after menses ; intense pain and enlargement of l. ovary—it could be seen protruding sausage-shaped—from which perceptibly was felt flatus passing downwards like small marbles, causing great pain, and discharging externally with a puff. 12.

Pain in groins (? ovaries) all day; slight leucorrhœa. 3 (10).

⁰Pain in uterine region, passing down inside of thighs, half-way to knees, and right leg feels numb. 26.

*Pains in *uterine region, all day, having no particular direction except down inner side of thigh half-way to knees. 1a 15.

Pains in uterine region. and particularly in region of l. ovary, extending down into thigh, uterine pains relieved by leaning back. *Pains intermittent. (*c. Veg. Lac. Lyc. Thuj.*) 1a (16).

Burning sensation in whole uterine region, also the ovaries. (*C. veg. Lach. Lyc. Thuj.*) (13, 14).

⁰Inflammatory and congested condition of uterus, with extreme soreness and tenderness, that made every motion, position, and even breath, painful. (***Bell***). 12.

⁰Rousing up and strengthening of uterus, bringing rapidly forwards the conditions preceding menses, which had formerly been dilatory and lingering for weeks. 12.

830. ⁰Sharp lancinating pains like knives (*Murex*) cutting upwards from os uteri, and as these were being relieved, sensation as of needles darting upwards in uterus. 12.

Congestion, redness, and extreme tenderness of os uteri, intensely aggravated. (by 75 m). 56.

*At sundry times during proving, an escape of flatus

from vagina. (*Brom. Lyc.*, *Nux. mos.*, *Nux vom.*, *Sang.*) 1.

Pressure on anterior part of vulva, entire relief by sitting; sensation as if everything were coming out at vulva. (*Apis. Lil.*, *Lyc.*, *Natr.*, *Sep.*, *Tarant*). 1d (7). (After 75 m).

°Bearing down as though everything would fall out through vagina. with very frequent desire to urinate, and smarting in urethra. 36.

The labia feels very much contracted, as from astringent applications. (*Cact.*, *Murex.*, *Nat. mur*). 1e (209 to 216). (After c. m).

°Great irritation about vulva and rectum. Diphtheria. 19.

Painless nodosity in upper part of r. labia, as large as a pea. 1e (256).

Pain in l. side of vulva. neuralgic in nature, short sharp; followed by slight discharge of blood from vagina several hours afterwards. 1e (34).

Very severe darting pains, passing from l. external labia through uterus to r. ovary, (*Bell.*, *Phos.*, *Thuj.*) continuing about two hours, and followed by a profuse discharge of bright-red blood; when the discharge ceased, (which was immediately after putting the feet in cold water), sharp burning pains were felt in r. ovary and r. temple; these pains very soon disappeared, but were followed by pains in l. ovary and l. temple; the pains alternated, first r. then l., lasting about an hour, when she fell asleep. 1e (8) (after C.M.)

840. *Itching in l. side of labia, with rough eruptive condition on l. side of vagina, with acrid leucorrhœa; excoriatng severely. 71 (12.)

°Great swelling of l. labia, and terrible pain while urinating; from gonorrhœa. 26 (after c. m.)

Pain in l. vulva, relieved by a slight discharge of blood 1a (12) (after c. m.)

Slight excoriation and itching of external labia. 1a (7).

*Itching of vulva. 1a (8). 1d (11).

Intense painful *soreness of vulva, extending to anus, coming on very suddenly about noon, and lasting for about two hours; came on again during evening;

could not *walk, *stand or *sit; relieved by *lying on the back and separating *the knees as far as possible. 1c (20).

Strong pulsations in vulva and vagina at various times during the proving ; and at such times, *great pain in vulva while sitting. (*Alum.*, *Murex*). 1e.

Intense itching of labia at night ; feels at times as if caused by something alive in it. (*Calad. Tarant.*) 1e (209 to 216).

°Parenchymatous metritis. (2 cases) ; in one, uterus 3 times as large as natural, round as a ball, and the body very hard, cervix obliterated by altered form of body; uterus sensitive. 32.

Intense itching and excoriation of external labia. (1-7).

Frequent desire to urinate, passing only a small quantity, causing intense burning and smarting as if there was a canker sore; this passed away before she had an opportunity to examine the parts; subsequently an induration appeared on inside of r. thigh, having a flat centre, like a pimple with the head cut off; this speedily increased to a large boil, the indurated part being near 3 inches in diameter, much inflamed, the top purple, and a small disk of pus under outer cuticle ; accompanied by chills, sweat, and general discomfort, while the extreme pain prevented sitting or lying with comfort. 1f (152).

850. *Raw and bad-smelling sores between labia and thighs, in the folds of the skin ; worse when walking, would rather keep still all the time ; these sores are covered with a disgusting white exudation. 1e (209 to 216).

Painful pimples on mons veneris. 1d (20).

Sexual organs extremely excited; very much increased from the slightest touch, as putting the hand on the breast, or from the pressure on the vulva when sitting, or the slight friction caused by walking. (*Cinnam.*, *Coff.*, *Lach.*, *Mosch.*, *Murex.*, *Plat.*) 1e (3).

° After-pains very distressing, extending to thighs, rather worse on r. side. 26.

°After-pains, very severe, and shooting down into thighs, 26.

°Several cases of retroverted uterus. 12.

°A great remedy for women, especially after miscarriage. 26.

°Menses very stringy and sticky, cannot get rid of them. 15.

°Much pain before and after menses, with severe headache and entire prostration for first day or so. °Parenchymatous metritis. 32.

°Menses nearly ceased; at menses much pain in r. thigh and uterus, constant desire for stool, very low-spirited. °Parenchymatous metritis, 32.

860. °Constant burning pain in left ovarian region, extending from l. leg even to foot. °Ovaralgia. 68.

°A serious case of uterine hemorrhage which had lasted with varying degree for 6 weeks, and had been treated "regularly" with no relief; the ovarian pains alternated sides, as did the chronic headache. 200th relieved hemorrhage permanently. 73 (per letter to me).

Flow not so profuse, nor so free as usual, but feels lighter and is better than usual at such times; on second day of menses, feet burned and face became hot and flushed, in two hours afterwards becoming cool and of a yellowish color. 3 (2).

*Urination caused intense pain in vulva, when even the least drop of urine comes in contact with it. 1a (8).

Menses four days too soon, otherwise normal. 1e (234).

*Discharge of blood from vagina twelve days after last menses had commenced, no pain. 1e (246).

MAMMAE.

Breasts very sore and sensitive to pressure, for a day or two during menses. 1e (319).

°Breasts very sore and painful, with sharp darting pain in r. ovarian region extending downwards to knee, very painful and must keep leg flexed: First day after miscarriage at sixth month. 26.

Pain in upper and outer part of breasts. 1a (34).

870. *Constant pain in breasts, they feel very sore when going up or down stairs. 1a (36).

*Breasts seem very full. 1a (35).

*Constant pain in nipples. 1a (35).

*Breasts sensitive to deep pressure. (*Calc.*, *Merc*, *Murex.*) 1c (6).

*Breasts painful to deep pressure. 1c (20).

*Breasts painful to slight pressure. 1c (19).

*Breasts very painful and sore; feel as if full of very hard lumps, very painful when going up or down stairs. (*Bell.*, *Calc.*, *Carb. au. Lyc.*, *Nitr. ac.*, *Phos.*) 1a (37).

*Breasts very sore and painful. 1a (38).

*Breasts very painful, but no lumps; the pains are caused by the least jar; has to hold the breasts firmly when going up or down stairs; breasts worse towards evening, so that the pressure of her arm, in its natural position, caused considerable pain. 1a (38).

*Breasts very sore, sensitive to the least pressure; dull constant, aching pain in them all the evening. (*Calc.*, *Murex.*) 1a (74).

880. Sore spot on r. side of r. breast, about the size of a silver dollar; very sensitive to touch, or to the jar caused by going up and down stairs; in three days, a similar sore spot on l. side of r. breast. 1a (57).

°Soreness and enlargement of breasts. (*Bell.*, *Bry.*, *Calc.*) 12.

°Loss of milk while nursing, without known cause. 12.

°Galactorrhœa. (Many cases). 12.

Dries up the milk when nursing. (*Puls.*) 12, 26, 33.

After weaning baby, r. breast full and painful, especially hard and painful on inner side; cannot bear her stays to press on it; it would feel very heavy if she had no stays on. 15.

°Knots and cakes in breast, after miscarriage. 1 (10m).

°Given for an ulcerated throat to a nursing woman, it cured the throat and nearly dried up the milk. 12.

°After CM (two doses) rapid decrease in size of breasts and quantity of milk in a lady who wanted to wean her child. 12.

Larynx and Trachea.

°Loss of voice. 33.

890. Voice perceptibly roughened, as if about to become hoarse. 40 (4).

Voice sounds changed; is very rough. 1a (5).

°Voice hoarse; interrupted by weakness and hoarseness. θDiphtheria. 20, 26.

Slight *hoarseness, with now and then a change of voice, after waking, but soon passing away. 44 (4).

°Hoarseness, child cannot cry aloud. 26.

°Excessive hoarseness, and tickling, choking sensation, relieved by moving about. 26.

°Respiration hoarse, crying was whispered and broken, often no sound at all. θDiphtheria. 22.

°Cough and dyspnœa. 23.

Frequent inclination to cough, from a tickling sensation in upper anterior part of larynx; worse in the house and while talking. 1a (7).

At 1.30 p. m., *tickling sensation in throat causing cough; in afternoon quite hoarse. (*Nitr. ac.*) 3 (6).

900. Cough from tickling in upper anterior part of larynx, worse *when tálking and also when lying down. 1a (10).

Cough from tickling sensation. 1a (11).

Cough from tickling in pharynx. 1a (12).

Dry hacking cough. 1a (13, 14, 17, 19.)

Cough from tickling in throat. 1a (22).

°Cough caused by irritation in upper part of throat, worse by laying down at night, also after eating and drinking, and during and after talking; with soreness of l. side of throat and constant desire to urinate. 20.

°Cough on taking a long breath, not when swallowing. 14.

°Hard metallic cough. 19.

Cough from tickling under middle of sternum. 1a (37).

Cough with pain and oppression of chest; it jars her all over. (*Rumex.*) 1a (37).

910. Considerable expectoration of slightly viscid mucous. 1a (3).

°Expectoration of profuse, thick, tough, white mucous in masses, with coryza. 14.

°Constant cough, accompanying soreness. θDiphtheria. 9.

°Constriction in lower part of larynx, like a finger across throat. 26.

°Larynx sensitive to pressure. θDiphtheria. 9.

Menses preceded by a dry, shaking, continuous cough, aggravated by speaking, caused by a dryness in larynx, and causing soreness in abdomen; this cough generally preceded menses and ceased after them; menstruation closed, with the blood, when wet being grass-green, drying dark-green. 1b (152 and subsequently).

°Voice hoarse and husky. °Diphtheria. 46.

°Unable to speak loud; distressed feeling while speaking. °Parenchymatous metritis. 32.

About 2 p. m., subsequent to the tightness of chest, very severe dry cough commenced; next day, dry hacking cough all day, with occasional severe paroxysms, very fatiguing, with cold hands and perspiration after coughing; in evening, after a hard spell of coughing, raised a little blood-stained mucous, a pinkish stain; no cough during night; laughing, or *talking seems to excite cough, she coughs almost continually while giving these symptoms; the sensation which provokes coughs is a soreness, fulness, and a sensation as if something might give way, and she would have hemorrhage; fears it; this same sensation extends through chest to lower inner angle of l. scapula; chest feels tired and sore: every cough hurts her half-way down sternum; feels as though the windpipe was peeled inside; the cough and soreness continue obstinate for several days, finally subsiding gradually under *Bellad.* 200. 63 (9)

°Croupy cough. °Diphtheria. 64. 32.

920. °Loss of voice, cannot speak in a whisper. °Pharyngitis. 12.

°Throat troubles her much if she reads aloud or talks more than usual; it seems almost as though it were stopping up, and she feels very hoarse, but has no soreness; there is a feeling of fulness and a sense of choking. 15.

°Marked soreness on touching larnyx. °Diphtheria. 32.

°Croupy cough, a dry hoarse bark, penetrating through closed doors all over the house. °Diphtheria. 32.

CHEST.

°Difficult breathing; during evening had several suffocating spells; mother feared she would die before I came. °Diphtheria. 25.

°Terrible dispnœa immediately after sleep, first on l. side of chest; the dispnœa compelled her to be lifted upright with violent exertion to get breath; there was sharp pain in region of heart with each of these attacks; after the medicine, had but one attack of dispnœa, and all the pain was referred to r. side of chest. °Acutc rheumatism. 14.

Lungs feel as though fast to chest, worse while writing. 43.

°Breathing hoarse and croupy, and at times an entire stoppage of breath, when it would resume with a violent effort. °Diphtheria. 14.

°Breathing often snoring, and only possible through mouth. °Diphtheria. 14.

Sighing frequently. 40 (3)

°Short breath. °After diphtheria. 25.

930. °Great difficulty in breathing, so he could not lie down flat. 19.

°Breathing very labored; could hear him breathe as you came upstairs. 19.

°Loud snoring during sleep. (Two cases). 25.

°Sensation as if the breath would leave her when lying down and trying to sleep; has to jump up and stir around for an hour or so every night. (*Grindelia robusta.*) 26.

After dinner, oppressed for breath, and has pain in upper part of lungs, shooting downwards. 3a (7)

Woke up just before daylight, feeling almost suffocated; had to go to the open window. 1a (6)

Oppressed for breath all day, only comfortable while in open air. *Puls.* 1a (6)

Sharp pain under fourth rib on r. side, when taking a deep inspiration. 1a (13)

Pain under fourth rib of r. side, when taking a long breath. 1a (14)

Soreness from r. clavicle down to third or fourth rib, worse on moving, less on l. side. 43.

940. Clavicles sore to touch. 43.

Right clavicle feels as if out of place, worse by moving shoulder 43.

Sore spot just to right of mid-sternum, worse from lifting or from pressure. 43.

Stabbing pain in r. lung, just below nipple, preceeded by pain in stomach-pit as of a stone or undigested food, at 9.45 p. m. 4 (1)

Stitches in r. lung on a line with nipple, aggravated by respiration. 12.

Severe pleuritic pain in region of fourth rib of r. side, much increased by prolonged inspirations. 1e (7).

Pain at the right fourth rib, very severe, so as to cause exclamations. 1e (8)

Severe pain in r. side in the deep muscles, worse from the least motion, especially from turning body to l. side; pain something like pleurisy, yet unlike it, not effected by respiration, yet made worse by taking off the corsets, as it then seemed to allow of greater motion of the parts: this lasted three days. 1e. (July 1872.)

Bruised sensation in r. side of chest when taking a deep inspiration. 1a. (20)

Pain in evening in region of seventh and eighth ribs of r. side, caused by deep inspiration. 1a (41).

950. During evening pain in region of seventh and eighth ribs during deep inspiration. 1a. (45, 51)

Sharp pain through l. lung forward. 4 (6)

Sharp neuralgic pain under nipple of l. breast, for one-half hour. 7 (5)

Whole l. chest feels sore and congested, could scarcely draw a long breath. (*Calc.*, *Ran. bulb.*, *Stann*). 1f (August, 1873).

Trembling sensation through chest and arms. 4 (7) (See Generalities.)

Trembling nervousness through chest, with sensation of uneasiness. 4 (10.)

Pain in chest and throat. 2 (10)

Soreness through chest to back. 43

Cramped feeling in chest, wants to stretch up and back. 43

Sore across mid-chest during forced expiration, feels just as if she had been struck. 43.

960. Boring pains in all parts of chest. 1f (August, 1873.)

Sharp pain in r. breast at 4 p. m. 2 (8)

Sharp pain like a stab in l. breast at 7 p. m. 2 (8, 9)
Chest quite sore in a line across nipples. 2 (10)
At noon, pains in upper chest, lasting the rest of day. 44 (5)
Raw sensation in chest as if it had been scraped. 1a (2)
Feeling of oppression and tightness behind sternum, with desire to draw a deep breath. 3 (42)
Dyspeptic aching pain behind lower end of sternum. 4 (15)
Fine stinging pain at middle of sternum; very superficial, lasting half an hour, but returning during evening. 1a (12)
Palpitation of heart, irregular, causing shortness of breath. 1c (7).
970. Sharp pain over apex of heart, for five minutes. 7 (1).
°Pulse so rapid it could scarcely be counted. °Diphtheria. 16.
°Pulse 130. °Tonsillitis. 16.
Pulse *quick, full and strong, with pain in chest and throat. 2 (10)
°Pulse of little volume. °Diphtheria. 17
°Pulse 130, wiry, weak. 19.
°Pulse quick and feeble. °Diphtheria. 9
*Pulse 100. 41 (3) °Diphtheria. Dyspepsia. 25
°Pulse 120. °Diphtheria. 25, 51, 46, 21.
°Pulse 140. °Diphtheria. 19, 23, 25, 12.
980. °Pulse 170. °Diphtheria. 22.
°Pulse 130-140. °Diphtheria. 23.
°Pulse almost gone. °Diphtheria. 12.
°Pulse 117. °Diphtheria. 48.
°Pulse, rapid, quick. °Acute rheumatism. 52.
Pulse 90 (with fever and diphtheretic throat) 62 (5)
°Heart beats rapidly from slight causes. °Parenchymatous metritis. 32.
°Respiration 21. °Diphtheria. 48.
°Difficult to breath at times. °Parenchymatous metritis. 32.
°Trembling, jerking, and fluttering through lungs, with numb, prickling sensation all over the body, legs, and arms. 26. (See Legs.)
990. Great difficulty of breathing, with increase of former sensation that throat was closing. 53. (1).

Sensation as of a hand in upper part of chest, or *lower part of neck; this tightness is very bad, afterward cough commenced. 63 (9).

Difficult breathing; could not get a full breath. 53a.

Oppression at chest; almost a soreness. 53b.

Sharp pain in r. side, a little in front; about the fourth rib, like a pleuritic stitch. 1.

Sharp pains in r. side. 1a (38).

Oppression and sense of suffocation in chest, similar to that experienced on sixth day of first proving; relieved by a dose of 10M. 1e (546).

°Paralytic symptoms strongly marked; as soon as he went to sleep, would stop breathing, and was only kept alive by keeping him awake; apparently respiration was kept up by voluntary effort. °Diphtheria. 75.

Authority: J. A. Wakeman, M. D.

BACK.

Pain in back, just below r. scapula. 1a (22, 33).

Pain in back below r. scapula. 1a (37, 40, 43).

1000. Sharp neuralgic pain under r. scapula. 7 (2).

Lameness and cutting pain under l. scapula, felt most when turning in bed. 4a (8).

Lameness through body from under l. scapula forwards, felt keenly at 7 a. m. 4a (9).

Sharp pain in l. scapula, for about three minutes. 3 (8).

Slight darting pain under l. scapula. 7 (1).

Sharp cutting pain under l. scapula, shooting forwards through lung. 4a (2).

Sharp cutting pain under l. scapula, shooting forwards through lung, with a similar pain under r. scapula, when lying turned partly towards the r. side and partly on back. 4a (3).

At 7.30 a. m., sharp cutting pain near l. scapula, as from rheumatism, worse on drawing a long breath; at 11.30 a. m., stitch in l. breast, very marked. 4 (5).

Piercing pain under l. scapula, running through the body. 4a (19).

Piercing pain under l. scapula, running through the body; felt keenly when turning in bed. 4a (28).

1010. Sweat on back while walking, though the day was very cold; after entering a warm room it chilled her through: thermometer at zero. (*Led. Petrol. Phos. Rhus. Sep.*) 1 (Dec. 25).

⁰Sharp incisive pain between scapulæ, passing through to sternum, with a sense of pressure or constriction of chest, in afternoon. 27.

Pain in back from scapulæ to sacrum. 1c (6).

Slight pains in scapulæ while sitting. 3 (6).

Backache between and just below scapulæ, when leaning forwards. 1a (17).

Backache nearly all day between scapulæ, worse after becoming warm, somewhat relieved by leaning back. 1a (5).

Backache between scapulæ. 1a (6, 8, 15).

Pain between scapulæ when leaning forwards. 1a (16).

Backache between scapulæ and in sacrum. 1a (20).

During evening, pain in back between scapulæ and in sacrum. 1a (38).

1020. ⁰Aching pains in all the limbs and back. ●Diphtheria. 36.

⁰Neck stiff. ●Rheumatism, neuralgic headache; ●Diphtheria. 25.

Pain in sacrum. 1a (13).

Pain in sacrum, increased by riding, not by walking. 1a (14).

⁰Pain in back of neck. ●Diphtheria. 9.

Aching pain in sacral region in morning, worse by stooping, relieved by leaning back, with a sort of weakness and giving away as if she would fall; this pain extended around l. side of pelvis (leaving the back) to inside of thigh, followed by a bloody leucorrhœal discharge after six hours, which came all at once, leaving labia extremely sensitive. 1f (152).

●Wandering pains in nape with stiffness. ●Rheumatism. 25.

⁰Backache. ●Diphtheria. 12, 17, 21, 51.

⁰Entire spine sensitive. ●Parenchymatous metritis. 32.

⁰Heat, pain, and beating in small of back. ●Parenchymatous metritis. 32.

1030. ⁰Neck aches, making her desire to bend head forwards. ●Parenchymatous metritis. 32.

⁰Wakes with severe pain in lower part of back, and it is often five minutes before she can straighten herself; this pain leaves her when she has been about

her work a short time, not returning till next morning. °Nervous throat affection. 15.

°Pain in back. °Diphtheria. 17, 21.

Pain and stiffness up r. sterno-cleido-mastoideus. 43.

In morning, began to feel painful fulness in back, across region of kidneys, much increased towards night; on lying down at night the pain ceased, also pains in calves, but returned soon after beginning to move next morning, continuing all day. 62 (4).

Sometimes darting pain in region of r. kidney. 62 (5).

°Spine aches from base of brain to coccyx. °Pharyngitis. 12.

Slight enlargement of already enlarged lymphatics in side of neck. 44 (11).

°Intense unbearable pain across super-sacral region, extending to r. natis and down r. sciatic nerve; the pain was so severe as to prevent sleep or rest; at sametime diphtheretic sore throat on r. side, with sensation of a lump, could not swallow solid food. 12.

UPPER EXTREMITIES.

Painful swelling and hardness, with suppuration, of l. axillary gland; menses came on at same time. 1e (195).

Sharp pain passing from r. shoulder to second joint of third finger. 1a (15).

1040. Pains down r. arm and in fingers, which feel cramped; does not seem to have the same power in r. hand. 43.

°From draught in evening, sudden violent pains in r. shoulder, so much so that when retiring that night she could not raise arm to finish toilet, as if disabled by dislocation. 25.

Pain in bend of r. elbow. 1a (20).

Tingling in r. forearm extending from elbow to little finger (*Arsen.*, *Con.*, *Merc.*, *Puls.*, *Sec.*,) at 10. a. m.; at 1.45 p. m., the same tingling, and with it the same sensation across r. calf, and a neuralgic pain in r. temple. 4 (2).

Right wrist lame and painful, (*Ox. ac.*, *Petrol*). 1a (13).

Severe pain for all of one day in r. wrist, pain seemed to be deep in centre. 1e (June, 1872).

Steady pain in r. hand as if it had been bruised. 3a (21, 22).

Pain in r. hand, passing from thumb to little finger. 1a (21).

Pain in ball of r. thumb. 1c (19).

Sharp shooting pains in ball of r. thumb. 1a (30).

1050. Pain in third finger of r. hand, extending from middle joint to tip. 1c (7).

Blotches looking like flea-bites on l. arm and both legs, which itch slightly; blotches had passed away next day. 3 (5).

Slight lameness of l. shoulder. (*Lach.*) 1a (9, 10).

Severe pain in metacarpo-phalangeal joint of index finger of l. hand, worse from pressure, also from bending the finger backwards; lasted severely about a week, but still continues a little (Nov., 1872). Severe pain of similar character in l. shoulder joint, felt only during certain movements of arm, especially when rotating it outwards or backwards (Nov. 20th, 1872); still continues (Feb., 1873); the same in both shoulders, with constant desire to urinate (March, 1874). 1e, 1f.

°Partial paralysis of l. arm, unable to raise hand to head; on attempting to do so was seized with sharp pains in arm below shoulder. 27.

Sharp pain round l. arm, as of a cutting instrument: felt principally at the vaccination-cicatrix; passed from thence to l. elbow and dissappeared. 4 (45 minutes after first dose).

At 8 p. m. sharp pain in upper part of l. arm, for about two minutes; then in the wrist. 3 (10).

Severe fine pain, lancinating in character, along outer border of l. biceps, worse when raising arm; this alternated with a similar pain in top of l. knee, which made it difficult to stand on the foot, and caused her to walk lame; at no time did the pains occur simultaneously; sometimes they would last 5 or 10 minutes in arm, and then all would go to knee, or they would last half an hour in one place and not go to the other; was scarcely free from for two days; never had them before or since. 1e (217, 218).

Severe pain in l. elbow. 1d (1).

Pain in l. elbow. 1d (2, 3).

1060. °Trembling of l. hand, as in paralysis agitans. 14.

Woke in night feeling very chilly, with *sharp pain in l. hand, and *sensation in left arm as if it was asleep ; lasting 15 minutes. 3a (9).

Palms and soles burning hot. 40 (3)

Palms grew hotter, and finally itched so frightfully that she could do nothing but sit and grind them together ; under their thick cuticle were numerous dark red macula as if an exanthem were about developing, and were only held in check by the horny epithelium. Palms abnormally hot to touch. 40 (5): hands still burn. (8).

°Two warts on little finger noticed to be leaving. 14.

Painful eruption in axillæ, like moist herpes, exceedingly painful on washing them. 1c (25, 26).

Herpetic eruption in both axillæ, with slight brownish scabs, extremely painful when washing them. 1e (7).

Herpetic eruption in both axillæ, mostly in r. with light brownish scabs, extremely painful when washing them. 1e (33).

Veins in hands look bluer than usual, they are swollen. 43.

Itching miliary eruption on both upper arms, continuing some time. 1e (Oct. 1872).

1070. Sensation as if an insect were crawling on shoulders and neck, occasionally on the hands. (*Nat.*, *Carb.*, *Nitr.*, *Phos. ac.*, *Secale.*, *Tabac.*) 1e (15 to 80).

Crawling sensation on shoulders, commencing just over or back of joint, passing up towards neck and up to edge of dress, as if a large insect were leisurely crawling in an indirect course; the sensation is so well defined that frequent fruitless examinations were made to find the insect. 1e (June to August 1872).

Fingers extremely cold, but not the rest of hand. *Cicuta.*, *Deflora.*, *Rhod.*, *Tarax.*) 1a (6) 1f (22).

Perspiration in axillæ, stains the linen bright orange-color, no smell. *Dulc.*, *Hep.*, *Nit. ac. Rhod,*, *Selen.*, *Sep.*, *Sulp.*, *Tellur.*, *Thuja.* 1 (Oct. 1872).

*Very fetid perspiration in axillæ, staining the linen brown. 1c (16).

*Fetid perspiration in axillæ. 1c (17).

Biceps very sore at lower part, only felt during motion, not from touch. (*Fluor. ac.*) 1a (41).

Wrists lame, (*Nux.*, *Kali.*, *Ruta.*) 1a (11, 21, 25, 40).

Wrists very lame, especially the r., which has sharp pains passing from thumb to little finger. 1a (12).

Wrists very lame. 1a (14).

1080. Wrists and knees lame. 1a (10).

Wrists lame and painful, especially r. 1a (20).

Aching in both wrists, especially when lifting anything. 1e (39 to 44).

Pains in all parts of both hands. 1e (12).

Pains in the hands. 1e (15, 18).

Soreness of ends of all the fingers for several days. 1f (August, 1873).

°Pain in one or the other shoulder. °Rheumatism. 25.

°Neuralgic pains in shoulders, left then right; then *vice versa.* 57.

°Shoulders and arms ache. °Parenchymatous metritis. 32.

°Left hand bloats and is numb, with trembling, jerking, and fluttering through lungs ; numb pricking sensation all over body, arms and legs. 26.

1090. Feels as if she wanted to fix shoulder so it would not feel strained. 43.

°Pain in l. shoulder extending across to r. L. worse, could scarcely move the arm. Pharyngitis. 12.

°Burning of hands and feet at night. °Ovaralgia. 68.

Lower Extremities.

A few days before menses, the inside of both thighs became raw and painful when walking, they then broke out with large, flat red pimples, no pus in them; the soreness soon left; but the pimples remain, they have no sensation. 1e (142).

During menses, the same pimples on thighs have come out; she worries herself for fear they will prove to be little snakes and twine and twist around each other. 1e (172).

The pimples return, and itch terribly. 1e (209 to 216).

°Partial paralysis of r. leg, from miscarriage; has to use a cane; r. ovary sore by spells, and pain darts down leg, sometimes to foot ; leg feels numb and stiff but cannot keep it still any length of time; feels better by flexing it on abdomen. 26.

Varicose veins on outer r. thigh, from hip to knee. 1d (3).

Severe pain in r. gluteal muscles; seems to catch her when she walks, so that she must bend to the r. and walk lame. 1 (Jan. 1873).

Sharp pain in upper part of r. thigh, during severe coryza. 3 (4).

1100. When walking, sensation of a pea on outer part of r. knee-joint, walks as if lame. 1e (7).

Sensation in right knee-joint as though the leg below were turned outwards; constant inclination to put the hand down and bring it into place again; felt only during evening: there was no displacement. 1e (138 to 160).

Pain in r. popliteal space. 1a (13 14).

Pain passing from r. popliteal space to back part of ankle. 1a (15)

Pain in r. popliteal space, relieved by stretching the limb out, and everting the foot. 1a (20) 1e (21).

Walks lame. 1a (20).

Right leg seems one or two inches too long. 1a (20).

Right leg feels longer than l. 1a (21).

Sharp lancinating pain in middle front of r. leg. 1e (545).

Fine sharp lancinating pain from middle of r. ankle in front, passing up leg about 8 inches, zigzag. 1e (293).

1110. Painful stitches in r. big toe when walking. 1a (10).

Pain in r. big toe when walking. (*Bry.*) 1a (11).

Knees and wrists lame 1a (10).

Rheumatic pains in l. hip and along sciatic nerve. θRheumatism. 25.

At noon, rheumatic-like pains in upper outer front of l. thigh. 44 (4).

Pain in inner and forepart of l. knee. 1a (20, 21).

Sensation of numbness in l. leg with great heat as if burning, but cool to touch; brought on by pressure on popliteal space, as on the edge of a chair; for two days. 1d (23, 24).

Sharp lancinating pains in l. ankle-joint internally, which causes immediate weakness, so that she would fall unless supported; lasts only for an instant. (*Nat.*, *Carb.*,) 1f (Feb. 1873).

After sitting awhile, on rising has an aching pain in top of l. foot, which prevents walking, and makes her fall; relief in a short time. 1c (545).

For about a week, whenever she rose after sitting awhile, has sharp pain in l. foot; passing from outside of heel to top of instep; for the first few steps she would have no control over the foot, and would walk as if lame; it would be felt again after sitting; would rapidly pass off. 1e (Nov. 1872).

1120. Burning of ball of l. big toe. 1a (26).

Burning of inner side of l. big toe. 1a (27).

°Temporary sciatica in l. thigh; said I had given him an opiate. 25.

Varicose veins on outside of both thighs; still visible on 126th day. (*Puls.*, *Psor.*,) 1e (4).

Sudden creeping chills in lower limbs. 1a (12).

Slight excoriation of skin between thighs, caused by walking. 1e (7).

Feeling of stiffness through thighs, nearly all day, worse on attempting to move after sitting. 3 (11).

Subject to attacks of acute rheumatism, and always had one after quinsy sore-throat. Bruised pain in soles, preventing walking, and a stiffness of ankle, knee, and hip-joints, and an occasional pain moving upwards; the pain became intense; she was confined to bed, and complained of pain in ankle-joints as of a dull plug pushing; joints were stiff and sore and tender to touch, with but little swelling; any application of fluid, whether cold or warm, made pain worse; worse from much heat and from least motion; then knees became involved, then hips and l. side of chest. At first l. ankle was attacked, then, after some hours suffering r. ankle, with relief to the part first affected; this would last two hours on r. side, and the pain would move back again to the joint first affected, and so the pain would see-saw from one side to the other, with relief in one side at a time; after 24 hours the joint higher up would be attacked, and the same programme be carried out. 14.

°Bruised pains in soles, making it difficult to walk; in

12 days the pains suddenly left the soles, and appeared in r. knee-joint, being smarting, lancinating, with light swelling of the joint; he could not move the affected limb, as the least motion increased the pains, as did also touch and the pressure of the bed-clothes. On the following day the l. knee-joint was affected in the same way, the r. becoming markedly relieved; but on the ensuing day, the r. was again affected, with relief to the l. Afterwards the hip joints were attacked alternately with the same symptoms which had affected the knee-joints; alternating like these in the pains and swelling, the l. joints being aggravated one day with relief of the r. and *vice-versa*, also lancinating pains appeared in the l. side of chest. After 4 days the wrist-joints were also affected, first the R. with the same symptoms as those of the lower extremities, the symptoms of one side of the body alternating with those of the other. He was not able to move himself in bed, the lancinating pains made him cry out continually: there was constipation, sleeplessness, but no fever; the pains and swelling were aggravated every evening, and especially by night, by movement, the effort to move himself in bed by touch and by the pressure of bed-clothes. 58.

1130. ⁰Articular rheumatism in r. hip and knee-joints, especially the former; she was seated in an arm-chair, unable to move, complaining of bruised, smarting, lancinating pains in both joints and in lumbar regions, with swelling of the effected joints; the pains aggravated by the slightest motion at night, by touch, and by the pressure of the bed-clothes. Next day the pains and swelling had gone to the l. hip and knee-joints, leaving the r. almost free: the ensuing day they had almost entirely disappeared from l. hip and knee-joints and had again attacked the r. hip and knee: there was complaining, moaning and sighing on account of her sufferings, and the termination of her illness. 58.

⁰The remedy *par excellence* for sciatica (*Curare*, *Graph*, *Graphal*, *Kali-bich*, *Lach.*, *Iris*, *Phyt.*, *Plaupn*, *Tallur.*) 1a.

Pains in the knees and wrists, *Ruta la.* (22)

In evening, pain in both knees; slight relief by stretching the limbs out straight. la (643).

Severe pain in front of both knees. 59.

Veins of feet and ankles very much swollen. le (12).

Feet swollen and very sore, causing considerable pain while walking. (*Eupat.*, *Pals.*, *Bry.*) la (7).

°Cramps in feet. (*Lyc.*, *Petrol.*, *Silic.*, *Sulp.*) 25.

°Ecthyma; a sore breaks out on r. leg, excessive itching causes by-and-by inflamation, then swelling, blisters forms and suppuration sets in; afterwards clear lymph, then discharge of matter; then scabs and scales will form, turning eventually into a bran-like desquamation; scars have left discolored skin. Case comes nearest to Neligan's *Atlas of Cutaneous Diseases*. Plate 3, fig. 2. 25.

Itching on calves, which, on being gently scratched, left a burning sensation; it extended up thighs, and on to the fleshy part of arms below elbows; most towards evening, and when warm: continued without redness or eruptions 14 days. 7 (15).

1140. Numbness and paralytic feeling in inner side of both knees, extending to both big toes. 60.

°Entirely disabled from walking or even standing. °Parenchymtous metritis. 32.

°Limbs cold to knees. °Diphtheria. 12.

°Pain in r. hip and leg while walking, with a trembling of the leg, and slight feeling of uncertainty, particularly on going down stairs. °Parenchymatous metritis. 32.

°Almost constant pain in r. hip. Parenchymatous metritis. 32

°Cannot walk any distance; trembling through r. thigh, and feeling as though entire lower portion of body was giving way; felt as though something were strained across lower part of bowels. °Parenchymatous metritis. 32.

°After exposure to cold night air when drunk; sharp darting pains, worse by any motion, with swelling in r. knee and r. ankle; next day joints of l. knee, l. ankle, l. hand, extremely painful, the same pain, moderately swollen, slightly red; ensuing day, l. ankle and knee better, but r. shoulder and elbow similarly affected: other joints unchanged in appearance. 52.

Pains in calves, (as well as the region of the kidneys) ceased on lying down at night, returning next morning soon after beginning to move. 62 (4).

⁰Can only walk with the assistance of a cane. ᶿHip-joint disease. 65.

Limbs very cold all night. 3 (45).

1150. Feet burn on 2nd day of menses. 3 (2).

FEVER.

Chilly feeling, lasting all day. 3a (10).

Internal chilliness, with external warmth. (*Arn.*, *Ars.*, *Bell.*, *Calc.*, *Cocc.*, *Dig.*, *Hell.*, *Iqn.*, *Lach.*, *Nux.*, *Sep.*, *Sil.*, *Thuja.*) 3 (51).

At 9.30 p. m., sudden chilly sensation, while the lips parch and burn. (*Arsen.*) 3 (17).

⁰Severe chills. ᶿDiphtheria. 17.

Cold and chilly all day till 4 p. m., when she becomes suddenly very warm, with *flushing of l. side of face. 1a (5).

At 4 p. m., felt very cold on entering house after being out of doors all day ; cold chills ran down back, and hands as cold as ice : at 6.30 p. m., entire relief after a hearty dinner. 3 (12).

*Slight rise of temperature. 41 (3).

Intense *fever on waking in morning, with perspiration. (*Eupat. Perf.*) 6.

⁰Fever, and bathed in warm perspiration, especially about face, neck and hands. ᶿDiphtheria. 22.

1160 ⁰Intense heat. ᶿDiphtheria. 16.

⁰Moderate fever. ᶿDiphtheria. 9.

⁰Fever. ᶿDiphtheria. 19, 31.

⁰Acute rheumatism. 52.

⁰High fever. ᶿDiphtheria. 12, 21, 25.

⁰Dry hot skin. ᶿDiphtheria. 23.

⁰Fever returning every afternoon. ᶿDiphtheria. 19.

⁰Temperature 102¾. ᶿDiphtheria. 16.

⁰Temperature 102. ᶿTonsillitis. 16.

⁰Temperature 103¼. ᶿDiphtheria. 48.

1170 ⁰Temperature 103. ᶿAcute rheumatism. 52.

⁰Sweat all over. ᶿDiphtheria. 20.

⁰Skin clammy. ᶿDiphtheria. 17.

⁰Exhausting sweats after sleep. 20.

°Fever and chills for a few days, and up and down every few hours. 19.

°Wakes in night in cold perspiration, with fearful forebodings. °Parenchymatous metritis. 32.

°Perspired considerably through night, sweat having a rank smell. °Acute rheumatism. 52.

°Sleep prevented by being very cold, for one hour after retiring with *great nervousness. 3 (16).

Woke in night feeling very chilly, with sharp pain in l. hand, and sensation in l. arm as if it was asleep, lasting 15 minutes. 3a (9).

*Feels feverish. 62 (5).

SLEEP.

1180. Very sleepy, could scarcely keep awake. 1a (3).

Very sleepy all day long, could scarcely keep awake, (*Sulph.*) 1a (20).

Very sleepy all day. 1a (21).

Sleepy during evening. 1a (6).

Very sleepy during evening. 1a (7, 19, 33, 40, 47, 58).

Can hardly keep awake in evening, even when reading something very interesting. (*Thuja*). 1a (209 to 216).

Goes to sleep in day-time if alone; would like to sleep even when people are around, but will not give up to it. 1e (209 to 216).

Sleep good; dreams pleasant, about statuary. 3 (4).

Sound sleep forepart of night; after 1 a. m., sleep broken and disturbed; uneasy fitful dreams till morning, the subject not remembered. 2 (3).

°Drowsy. °Diphtheria. 3.

1190. °Great desire to sleep. °Diphtheria. 12.

°Cried out and talked in sleep. °Diphtheria. 21.

°Sleeplessness from emotional strain, with entire nervous debility. 25.

*Cannot find any comfortable position in bed; there is no way she can put her hands that they do not bother her; falls asleep at last on her face. 1.

When in bed, the arms seem to be in the way somehow, cannot get them into a comfortable position; on waking, the hands are over the head. *Calc.*, *Chin.*, *Coloc.*, *Nux.*, *Plat.*, *Puls.*, *Rheum.*, *Ruta.*, *Thuja*, *Verat.*.) 1e (209 to 216).

Very restless at *night; very difficult to get into a comfortable position; generally go to sleep lying on back with hands over head. 1e (June, 1872),

Sleep broken and very bad. 2 (10).

*Sleep disturbed, very wakeful; limbs very cold all night. (45).

Began to be very restless at night, even in sleep; restlessness most marked when attempting to sleep, could not sleep until late at night: rolled and tossed about all night, could not sleep at all on account of uncontrollable feeling of restlessness; had to turn and shift about constantly; utter inability to lie half a minute in one position: the nightly restlessness lasted till 8th day. 40 (3).

*Very restless all night: could not keep any clothes over her. 1e (8).

1200 Extremely *restless at night, rolling and tossing about momentarily, sighing deeply. 42 (5).

All night *very restless, tossing about, moaning and groaning during sleep; next night, restless with hot hands and feet; but slept better than on previous night. 41 (2).

⁰Sleepless and crying continually. 26.

⁰Sleeps a great deal in day-time, and sleepless and crying all night long. 26.

⁰Very restless, cannot sleep much. ᶿParenchymatous metritis. 32.

⁰Very little restless sleep at night, bad dreams. ᶿParenchymatous metritis. 32.

Dreams of the events of the day, but much magnified. (*Bry.*, *Calc.*,) 1.

Dreams confused. 2 (2).

Dreams of going to the sea-shore or to the water many nights in succession. 1.

Dreams of pleasant interviews with friends. 4 (8).

1210. Sleep at night full of sensuous dreams, with conscious emissions. 44 (4).

Sensuous dreams at night, but no emission. 44 (4).

Very distressing dreams about cats. *Arsen.*, *Hyos.*, *Mez.*, *Puls.*) 1a (20).

Dreams of a very beautiful vision; as if the heavens opened and disclosed scenes of indescribable beauty. (*Stann.*) 1.

Continually dreams of eating all night, but does not dream that she is hungry ; dreams in connection of walking a great distance. 1e (245).

Dreams of eating to excess almost every night ; yet during the day not the least desire for food, though it tastes good when eating. 1e (April & May, 1872).

Dreams of seeing nice things to eat, and of having a great desire for them ; yet as soon as she eats, is terribly nauseated. 1

Dreams of eating, but everything nauseates her terribly ; it makes her sick to think of it, even when awake. 1.

Dreams of playing ghost, and going around to scare folks. 1.

Dreams of going home, and always getting into trouble ; of going to see people, and being disappointed because they were not glad to see her. 1.

1220. Dreams that she is naked in public streets, or other places, and feels terribly about it for awhile, and then consoles herself that, as she has an exquisitely beautiful form it will make no difference. 1.

Dreams frequently that she has a child, but that it has no father, and that she is disgraced by it ; she never dreams of its birth, only that it is hers some other way. 1.

Dreams of traveling great distances, but generally is in trouble, missing trains, boats, and stages. 1.

Dreams of going a journey, and was separated from the party, and had to walk a long distance, and arrived at the station just in *time to see the train start off. 1 (*Deflor.*, *Lach.*, *Sang.*, *Sil*).

Dreams of a terrible pain in l. side of chest ; felt as if her corsets were broken and sticking into her ; the agony was intense when taking them off : woke up exhausted. 1f (Aug., 1873.)

Dreams of vermin, especially bed-bugs, very distressing ; there seemed to be multitudes of them. (*Anem.*, *Carb.*, *Mur.*, *Ac.*, *Nux.*, *Phos.*) 1.

Dreamed that she was all one mass of sores inside of her, and that small round fat worms (like cheese maggots) were crawling out of the vulva, and going all over her ; she would take them off, yet more would come, and she would feel them crawl out one after the other, just as plain as if it were really the case: on waking, the sensation continued, with violent itching of vulva, but was afraid to touch it for fear that the sores in the groins had indeed generated worms. 1e (209).

Dreams of a visit from the devil (knew him by the appearance of his body, as seen through a rent in his clothes, which was as a glowing red-hot coal), who urged her to eat and drink divers articles; on her refusal, took her to his anatomical museum, where he had the hands of those who had pledged him, and the hearts of those who had bartered them for wealth, power and fame. (*Kali.*, *Nat.*, *C.*, *Niccol.*) 1.

Sleep very much disturbed by dreams; two or three times was witnessing blood-shed; also dreamed that she was lost in some old ruins, and could not find her way out. 39 (2).

°Dreamed a large snake was in the bed. θTonsillitis. 8.

1230. °Sleep restless. θNervous throat affection. 15.

Got to sleep late; profuse *sweat during sleep; felt feverish all night; in morning feels better in every way. 62 (4).

Dreamed that she had hemorrhage of lungs; caused by the bad feeling in lungs. 63 (9).

°At night lies with l. leg flexed on thigh, and thigh on pelvis; very restless all night, feels worse after sleep. θOvaralgia. (left side) 68.

Dreams frequently that she is *urinating, and wakes to find herself on the point of doing so, requiring immediate relief. 1.

Skin.

Every scratch gets sore. 43.

°On face, hands, neck and chest, bright scarlet eruption, exactly like scarlatina. θDiphtheria. 51.

°Bright scarlet redness on chest and round neck; next day extending all over body except legs, which were, however, covered that night; on this last and next day (5th and 6th days) when the fever and diphtheria were at their height, the skin in large patches assumed the dark red color bordering on purple, as seen in malignant cases, while the whole body seemed swollen. °Diphtheria. 21.

°Diphtheria with or following scarlatina. 20, 21.

°Icthyosis, with bran-like desquamation of skin. 12 (after Sulph. and Psor. had failed).

1240. °Several boils on l. side. °Sick headaches. 15.

°Crusts on skin, under which greyish yellow matter formed and was squeezed out. 32.

GENERALITIES.

*No inclination for the least exertion, would like to do nothing but sleep. 1e (209 to 216).

*Much lassitude. 2 (1).

Totters when walking, *tired. 43 (19).

°Heaviness, weakness, general languor. °After Diphtheria. 25.

°Profound depression of vitality. °Diphtheria. 9.

*General weakness and prostration very marked. 5.

Great exhaustion, with "poisoned" feeling. °Diphtheria. 20.

°Profound prostration, to the extent of refusing to make the effort to take a dose of medicine. °Diphtheria. 16.

1250. °In the morning so much prostrated that she could not turn in bed ; so tired. °Diphtheria. 51.

°Very weak. °Diphtheria. 12.

°Prostration turns; every two hours like sinking, in typhoid fever. °Diphtheria. 12.

°Unable to leave bed. °Parenchymatous metritis. 32.

°Sinking spells every morning, attended with great nervousness. °Parenchymatous metritis. 32.

°Often feels as if she would lose use of limbs. °Nervous throat affection. 15.

°Languid, strength giving out. °Diphtheria. 19.

°Much prostrated. °Diphtheria. 16, 21, 23.

Felt in fine spirits ; ran for nearly half a mile without fatigue. 4a (16).

°When walking, seems to be walking on air ; when lying, does not seem to touch the bed. (*Asar., Chin., Coff., Nat., M., Nux., Op., Rhus., Spig., Stram., Thuja.*) 22.

1260 Very nervous when trying to sleep. (*Apis, Phus.*) 3 (16).

Feeling of great uneasiness during forenoon; very nervous with trembling sensation through arms and chest. 4 (7)

^{0}Rheumatic pains in joints. 28.

General feeling of illness all day, but no return of diarrhœa. 44 (6).

Has improved remarkably in flesh, and promises to have her bones fairly cushioned with fat; never showed any tendency to fatten before the proving. 41.

Feeling very weak and depressed: went to bed at 8 p.m. from fatigue and indisposition; slept well till 9 a.m. 44. (7.)

Felt very unwell. 44 (11).

^{0}Feels ill. $^\theta$Diphtheria. 51.

Woke late, with tired feeling and inclination to lie longer in bed; better after dressing; remainder of day tolerably comfortable. 44 (12).

Indisposed all day, appetite poor. 44 (13).

1270. Woke earlier than usual; felt well till 3 p.m., unwell rest of day. 44 (17).

^{0}Restless, going from rocking-chair to lounge, back and forth. $^\theta$Diphtheria. 19.

^{0}Very restless, cannot stay indoors, and when out of doors cannot remain long in any place, runs all over town; feels best when walking in open air. 26.

^{0}Restless all over, head, legs, and whole body. $^\theta$Diphtheria. 20, 26.

^{0}Great restlessness over entire body. $^\theta$Diphtheria. 9.

^{0}Restlessness. $^\theta$Diphtheria. 17, 19, 21.

Utter inability to lie half a minute in one position. 40 (3)

^{0}Restless day and night. $^\theta$Parenchymatous metritis. 32.

^{0}Numb pricking sensation all over body, arms and legs. 26.

^{0}Pricking sensation over body, arms and legs. $^\theta$Diphtheria. 9.

1280. General aggravation at 5 p.m. $^\theta$Diphtheria. 9.

^{0}Rheumatism of legs and chest symptoms. 14.

^{0}Aggravation of symptoms after sleep. (*Kali-bich, Lach., Op., Stram., Sulph.*) $^\theta$Diphtheria. 16, 20.

The symptoms all through the proving have occurred

periodically; *worse morning of one day, and afternoon of next. 1

⁰Aggravation morning of one day, evening of next. ⁰Diphtheria. 9.

Feeling as if she had taken cold, but was confident she had not. 5.

A langour, a tired sleepy feeling during day; in fact, a longing to lie down; often this feeling of drowsiness is so overcoming that they get up from one lounge only to fall on their face on another; afterwards, usually increased appetite. 61.

⁰Symptoms better in evening, moderately quiet at night, but worse from about 4 a.m. to 7 a.m. ⁰Diphtheria.

⁰Neuralgia and acute pains; rheumatism, gout, syphilitic sciatica, sexual debility. 25.

⁰Chronic rheumatism alternating sides; much relieved. 14.

1290. The pains commence on either sides; they go from one side to the other; one side entirely recovering before the other is attacked. (See various symptoms given above).

⁰The pains are constantly flying from one part to another. *Puls.* 13.

⁰The characteristic is the erratic disposition of the symptoms. 45.

⁰Syphilitic rheumatism, pains shifting; aggravations at 5 p.m. and 7 a.m. ⁰Diphtheria. 14.

⁰Child prefers to sit up in its mother's arms, though weak. ⁰Diphtheria. 22.

⁰Sequelæ of diphtheria.

⁰Sequelæ of syphilis.

⁰Child partially paralyzed after diphtheria; could not walk; pain all over, with cough, aphonia, loss of appetite, emaciation. 29.

⁰The red, shining, glistening appearance is characteristic in any ulceration. 14.

⁰Enlarged glands after scarlatina. 18.

1300. ⁰Cold durations. 18.

Useful in scrofula. 18.

⁰Rachitie. (Allopathic authority.)

⁰Emaciation. 29, 33.

⁰Chiefly affects left side. 50.

Dioscorides, Rhasis, Pliny and Sextus recommend it for the removal of the dead foetus. Sammonicus and Sextus praise it in photophobia and otitis. Pliny claims that it cures ulceration of the internal os. It was considered an antidote to deadly poisons. (From C. H.)

°Pains all over as if in bones. θDiphtheria. 12.

Pains in limbs. 53 (1).

θDiphtheria. 17, 21.

°Pains in all the bones.

1310. θAcute rheumatism. 52.

°Many pains coming and going, and appearing now here, now there. θAcute rheumatism. 52.

°Follows *Lachesis* well. 26. Hg.

°Several cases cured resembled *Lachesis*. θDiphtheria. 20.

°Follows well when *Nitric Ac.* seems indicated, but fails to act. 14.

Concordance.

(1) *Lach*, *Lyc.*, *Thuja.*

(2) *Kali bich*, *Merc.*, *Nat. S.*, *Nit. Ac.*

Bellad. 200. Removed cough and soreness of chest. 63.

°After vomiting all day, had a rather severe faint in evening, and has felt weak and out of sorts ever since. θSick headache. 15.

°Pains in limbs as if they had been beaten. θPharyngitis. 12.

°Certain forms of colic, or acute pains in certain portions of the body, as well as sore throats, when the pain alternates from one side to the other at regular intervals. 69.

1320. °Pains and disorders *of all kinds* changing from one side to the other: first observed in diphtheria, if first one then the other tonsil was affected, changing repeatedly. 13.

°Since sick headache was cured, has had to procure clothing of larger size. 74. (Authority J. T. Kent, M.D.

ERRATA.

Page 4, line 25 for molecure, read molecule.
" 18, top, for Hycoph read Hypoch.
" 20, S. 352 ; for rotton, read rotten.
" " " 364 ; for vulvæ, read vulva.
" 22, " 405 ; for ovarion, read ovarían.
" 37, for Trifolia read Trifolium.
" 41, No. 40 ; for hypergastric, read hypogastric.
" " " 41 ; for membraneous, read membranous.
" " " " for diphtheretic, read diphtheritic.
" 47, S. 30 ; for puls., read Puls.
" 49, S. 70 ; for Strout, read Stront.
" " S. 74 ; for Ramex read Rumex.
" 51, S. 112 ; for Mix read Thuj.
" 52, S. 40 ; for Kalib, read Kali b.
" 54. S. 103 ; for Thus read Thuj.
" 57, S. 230 ; for Nitrogen, Protoxide, read Nitrogen protoxide.
" 60, S. 280 ; for ol. an., read Ol. an.
" 74, S. 486 ; for Jgnat, read Ignat.
" 77, S. 545; for Post Scarletina, read Post Scarlatinal.
" 78, S. 547; for Strout, read Stront.
" 79, S. 564 ; for Nat. Mur., read Nat. mur.
" 82, S. 632 ; for Sach. Alb., read Sacch. alb.
" 83, S. 647 ; for Nat. Nit., read Nat. nit.
" " S. 651 ; for Rau. bulb., read Ran. bulb.
" 86, S. 696 ; for foeces, read fæces.
" 90. S. 768 ; for glands, read glans.
" 93. S. 826 ; for C. veg., read C. veg.
" 94, for labia, read labium.
" 97, S. 876 ; for Carb. au., read Carb. an.
" 100, S. 923 ; for dispnœa, read dyspnœa.
" 107, S. 1070 ; for Nat. Carb., read Nat. carb.
" 110, S. 1117 ; " " " " "
" 111, S. 1131 ; for Graphal. read Gnaphal.
" " " for Plaupn, read Plant. m.
" " " for Tallur, read Tellur.
" " 1132 ; for Ruta la., read Ruta, l. a.
" 112, S. 1136 ; for Pals., read Puls.
" 113, S. 1152 ; for Iqn., read Ign.
" " S. 1158 ; for Eupat. Perf., read Eupat. perf.
" 116, S. 1225 ; for Mur. Ac., read Mur. ac.
" 117, S. 1227 ; for Nat. C., read Nat. c.
" 118, S. 1259 ; for Nat. M., read Nat. m.
" 119, S. 1260 ; for Phus., read Rhus.
" 121, S. 1310 ; for Lye, read Lyc.
" 121, S. 1310 ; for Nat. S., read Nat. s.
" 121, S. 1310 ; for Nit. Ac. read Nit. ac.